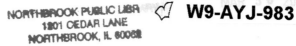

USMLE STEP 1
made ridiculously simple

Andreas Carl, M.D., Ph.D.
Adjunct Assistant Professor
University of Nevada School of Medicine
Department of Physiology and Cell Biology
Reno, NV 89557-0046

MedMaster, Inc., Miami

Notice: The author and publisher of this book have taken care to make certain that the recommendations for patient management and use of drugs are correct and compatible with the standards generally accepted at the time of publication. As new information becomes available, changes in treatment and use of drugs are inevitable. The reader is advised to carefully consult the instructions and information material included in the package insert of each drug or therapeutic agent before administration. The author and publisher disclaim any liability, loss, injury or damage incurred as a consequence, directly or indirectly, of the use and application of any of the contents of this book.

ISBN10 #0-940780-91-7
ISBN13 #978-0-940780-91-0

Made in the United States of America

Published by
MedMaster, Inc.
P.O. Box 640028
Miami, FL 33164

For Dr. Anna Ivanenko.

INTRODUCTION

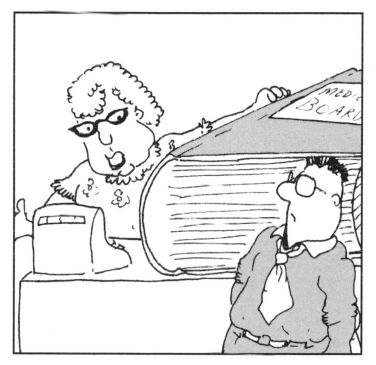

"This is the most complete book for the USMLE,
unfortunately no one can carry it out of the store."

FIRST OF ALL: FREE DOWNLOADS

Before you do anything else, please download a 1,000 QUESTIONS QUIZ and a list of IMAGE LINKS for the USMLE here:

www.medmaster.net

1,000 QUESTIONS QUIZ is in "mix and match style" and tied to the contents of this book. You should practice some clinical vignette style questions in the format given on the USMLE. However clinical vignettes are very inefficient for review of knowledge content, since you need to read a very lengthy question description just to test one single knowledge fact. The "mix and match" style allows you to test several items at once in a much shorter time. You probably will find these questions difficult and challenging. Once you have worked with this book for a while, it should get easier and easier.

IMAGE LINKS require a hookup to the internet. You will find the most important and relevant images for the USMLE Step-1 exam here. Many times a picture says more than thousand words. Please try them all!

PREFACE TO THE 6th EDITION

The USMLE Step-1 exam has become increasingly clinical in nature and it is more important than ever to be able to relate the basic medical sciences you have learned in med school to clinical case presentations (clinical vignettes). I have increased the amount of clinical correlations and placed each chart into a context. Hopefully, this will make "*USMLE Made Ridiculously Simple*" most useful as a study tool, in addition to being a great "memory aid".

Your score on the USMLE Step-1 exam not only depends on how hard you study, but also what you study. Obviously, if you study what they ask, you can achieve a very high score. I have prepared this manuscript in order to help you maximize your efforts. The material has been selected based on many years of teaching basic medical sciences to medical students and my own experience taking the USMLE exams. There have been significant changes in USMLE format and content and I wish to thank the many students whose input has allowed me to keep this book current and relevant for the USMLE exam.

Please visit my website to share your experiences with other students:

www.usmle.net

If you are about to take the exam or just took it, you can also contact me by e-mail:

andreas_carl@usmle.net

THE USMLE STEP-1 EXAM HAS BECOME SO CLINICAL IN NATURE, SHOULD I STUDY INTERNAL MEDICINE?

You will find that most USMLE exam questions are wrapped into clinical case presentations, but in the end you still will need to know the basic sciences in order to answer the questions. It is NOT necessary to know internal medicine to pass this exam (although it wouldn't hurt). Practically what this means for your test preparation is that you should focus on areas of basic sciences that have clear relevance to clinical medicine since these are much more likely to be made into a "clinical vignette" than some esoteric unconnected science facts. For this reason I have increased the number of clinical comments and explanations for the current edition of this book.

WHAT ARE HIGH-YIELD FACTS?

You need to know that what may be of high yield in one year could very well be of low yield the next year. There are some clear trends (emphasis on molecular biology, de-emphasis of gross anatomy) but with the random selection of questions by the testing computer, you cannot rely on "high-yield facts" alone. You must be able to place these into a practical context. The new edition of this book provides this context wherever possible. Many illustrations have been added to clarify concepts and to make the reading a more enjoyable experience.

WHAT THIS BOOK IS NOT:

Medical Boards Made Ridiculously Simple is not a textbook and I recommend you use it side-by-side with your other review books. I have tried to be clear, comprehensive and very brief. As you become more familiar with the material, you should be able to read through entire chapters within an hour or two and develop a feeling of "deja-vu" which is a good sign and means you are getting ready for the exam!

WHY THE CHART FORMAT?

Well, I made these charts for myself when I took the USMLE and found it a fantastic memory-aid! Charts allow a more logical arrangement of basic science facts that can easily be built upon rather than just a random collection of materials. Studying in such a systematic fashion lets you avoid the "high-yield trap". I have chosen the chart-format in order to provide the **maximum amount of information with the minimum amount of words**. By concentrating on key associations you will certainly improve your performance in multiple-choice situations.

HOW TO USE STEP-1 MADE RIDICULOUSLY SIMPLE?

This book is best used side by side with your other text and review books. You can personalize the charts by adding information that appears important or interesting to you. **The logical arrangement of basic science facts in charts will make it very easy to review all USMLE subjects just a few days before the exam**. I recommend reviewing the tables many times until they become boring. It's not necessary to be able to actively reproduce all material given here, as long as you recognize key associations in a multiple-choice situation. As usual, concentrate on the BASICS FIRST...!

> ➤ Use it during your course work to organize your thoughts
> ➤ Use this book as a **refresher course**
> ➤ Use this book as a **last minute review**
> ➤ Use this book as a **testing tool**

You can – and should !!! – use this book as a TESTING TOOL in a similar fashion like you would study vocabulary of a foreign language: Cover the right part of the chart with your hand, and check if you can recall the key features or key associations of each item:

1.15.) AUTOSOMAL DOMINANT DISEASES

familial hypercholesterolemia	abnormal LDL receptor coronary artery disease
familial polyposis	colon cancer
spherocytosis	hemolytic anemia
von Willebrand disease	...ng
Ehlers-Danlos syndrome	s... sp... ...ions
Marfan syndrome	long... lens...
achondroplasia	prema... dwarfis... ...al trunk
phacomatoses	benign tumo...
Huntington's disease	chorea dementia
polycystic kidney disease (adult type)	kidney failure

Some charts marked 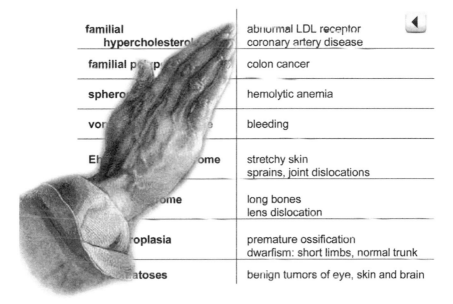 are also suitable for REVERSE TESTING: Cover the left part of the chart and ask yourself questions like:

- Which autosomal dominant disease is characterized by abnormal LDL receptors?
- Which autosomal dominant disease increases the risk of colon cancer?
- Which autosomal dominant disease causes hemolytic anemia?

…and so on… Ask your friends or study partners! Enjoy!

1.15.) AUTOSOMAL DOMINANT DISEASES

familial hypercholesterol	abnormal LDL receptor coronary artery disease
familial p...p...	colon cancer
sphero...	hemolytic anemia
vo...	bleeding
Eh...ome	stretchy skin sprains, joint dislocations
...ome	long bones lens dislocation
...oplasia	premature ossification dwarfism: short limbs, normal trunk
...atoses	benign tumors of eye, skin and brain

"Praying hands" borrowed from Albrecht Dürer.

PATHOLOGY

- Pathology should be the centerpiece of your studies; it is also the most valuable for your future practice of medicine. If you want to follow a pathology-centered approach to the USMLE, then get the *"Rapid Review Pathology"* (10) by Dr. Goljan, a most excellent review source.

- Robbins-Cotran's (1) is the top book in the field, but too long for review. If you have used it during your class you may want to review the pictures and highlighted texts. For USMLE review in outline format, the *Board Review Series Pathology* book by Schneider and Szanto (11) is highly recommended.

- Spend a day or two just looking at pictures, until you can recognize the most important ones (see *"High-Yield Pictures"* at end of chapter 1 of this book), but don't go overboard – in many cases you will be able to answer the question from the case presentation alone, even if you don't recognize the picture.

MICROBIOLOGY

- *Clinical Microbiology Made Ridiculously Simple* (12) is the number one best selling microbiology book in the US featuring over 200 cartoons which can make even this sometimes hard and dry subject easy and fun!

- Also check out Levinson's (13) well-renowned review book. It contains a highly crammable list of the medically most important species and great practice questions.

- Know all the details, structure/function of the HIV virus. Study therapy of AIDS related infectious diseases. High-yield topic!

- If you have time to spare, read *Immunology* from the Illustrated Review Series (14). There are many questions on the exam, and this book covers it all.

BIOCHEMISTRY

- Champe-Harvey (15) is "dead-on". If you know this book, you should get close to 100% right on the USMLE exam. Pay special attention of the last few chapters covering molecular biology, which is always very high-yield.

- In case you got lost, I recommend *Clinical Biochemistry Made Ridiculously Simple* (16) for a quick overview of the wondrous and amazing "Land of Biochemistry", including a topographical map of pathways.

PHARMACOLOGY

- Harvey-Champe (17) again is "dead-on". If you know this book well, you should get close to 100% right on the USMLE exam.

- *Clinical Pharmacology Made Ridiculously Simple* (18) contains a large number of tables comparing drugs side by side. Very useful and complete! Excellent review, not just for the exams but also for later.

- I found flash cards very useful for this subject. Make two sets: one for drug names versus mechanism of action and/or indication, and one set for drug names versus side effects! It is always best to make your own flash cards.

ANATOMY

- Don't spend too much time on this subject. Best preparation is to look at pictures, including plenty of cross sections (CT or MRI scans) of the body.

- Read *Clinical Anatomy Made Ridiculously Simple* (19), but even this may be overkill.

- Read *Clinical Neuroanatomy Made Ridiculously Simple* (20). Read this one twice!

- Embryology and Histology are very minor subjects.

PHYSIOLOGY

- A difficult subject because you cannot memorize it. Even if you knew your Ganong or Guyton (6), you may not be able to answer all questions. Linda Costanzo's review books are the most popular (21, 22).

- I personally like *Color Atlas of Physiology* by Silbernagel and Despopoulos (23) for a quick review. Most beautiful color pictures filled with large amounts of information.

- Look at charts and diagrams. Learn how to interpret these!

- A recent trend on the USMLE is receptors, signal transduction mechanisms and molecular biology of the cell. Learn as much about these important topics as you possibly can!

SOCIAL SCIENCES

Don't waste too much time here, but I recommend you read *BRS: Behavioral Sciences* from the Board Review Series (24). Some things you need to know very well are:

*   Differences between normal grief reaction and adjustment disorders, neuroses and psychoses, dementia and delirium.

*   Defense mechanisms.

*   Sensitivity / Specificity / Negative predictive value etc. It's not enough to memorize what to divide by what; you need to understand the meaning of these.

*   Ethical questions. Expect many clinical vignettes and scenarios asking you, what is the most appropriate thing to say as doctor. Be "politically correct", non-judgmental and ask your patient open-ended questions.

PRACTICE QUESTIONS

*   You will find the real exam very different from any collection of multiple choice questions or practice tests currently on the market. The real exam is more clinical in nature and questions tend to be longer. Don't panic - everyone is "in the same boat". There are retired board questions, but remember: they are retired for a reason! I found the *Pretest Questions* series very thorough but more difficult than the actual board exam. The *NMS Review for USMLE Step 1* questions (9) are a bit easier and their style matches the actual USMLE well. Practice as many questions as possible.

*   For Web resources, try either Kaplan or USMLE World. Both have a good reputation.

*   Don't use questions to "test" yourself. Don't be concerned about how many percent you get right. Mark all questions you get wrong, identify your areas of weakness and concentrate your studies on these. Later review just the questions you got wrong the first time and see how much you have learned.

*   Don't practice any multiple choice questions the week before the exam. You will get tired, bored and frustrated. Negative feelings might carry over to exam day.

ADVICE FOR FOREIGN MEDICAL GRADUATES

*   It's especially important to get a great score the first time around since it is becoming more and more difficult for foreign medical graduates to get into a Residency program. If you are IMG, just passing is not good enough! Aim high!

- Only 70% of foreign medical graduates pass on first attempt, compared to 95% of US or Canadian medical students. A major reason for this difference is language comprehension. Make sure you study from US review books since emphasis may be quite different from what you learned in your own country.

- Questions on the USMLE are sometimes exceedingly long and you may struggle to finish in time. Practice as many questions as you can (~ several thousand). Make sure to practice some under "real-time" conditions: do 60 questions in 1 hour without a break.

- Often it is useful to read the last sentence of each question first, then take a quick glance (no more!) at the answer choices, then go back and read the text of the question very selectively.

IMPORTANT

- Don't study any new material the day before the exam. It is more important to be well rested. For every fact you memorize on the day prior to the exam, you will lose some other facts!

THANKS

I wish to thank MedMaster for the beautiful cartoons and for permission to use illustrations from many of their other titles. Figures 4.29-4.38 were modified and reproduced with permission from Smith, L.H. and Thier, S.O. *Pathophysiology - The Biological Principles of Disease*. W.D. Saunders Co., 1985. Others as indicated.

I hope that this text will help your preparation for the USMLE Step 1 and would appreciate any comments about the selection and presentation of this material you might have. Good luck!

GOLD STANDARD TEXT BOOKS

These are the very best and will last you a lifetime as reference:

1. *Pathologic Basis of Disease*, Robbins, Cotran; Saunders
2. *Sherris Medical Microbiology*, Ryan et al., McGraw-Hill
3. *Pharmacological Basis of Therapeutics*, Goodman&Gilman; McGraw-Hill
4. *Lehninger Principles of Biochemistry*, Nelson, Cox; Freeman
5. *Gray's Anatomy - The Anatomical Basis of Clinical Practice*, Standring; Churchill Livingstone
6. *Textbook of Medical Physiology*, Guyton, Hall; Saunders
7. *Kaplan and Sadock's Comprehensive Textbook of Psychiatry*, Sadock et al.; Lippincott Williams & Wilkins

POPULAR REVIEW BOOKS FOR THE USMLE

8. *First Aid for the USMLE Step 1*, Le, Bhushan; McGraw-Hill
9. *NMS Review for USMLE Step 1*, Lazo et al.; Lippincott Williams & Wilkins

10. *Rapid Review Pathology*, Goljan; Mosby
11. *BRS Pathology (Board Review Series)*, Schneider, Szanto; Lippincott Williams & Wilkins

12. *Clinical Microbiology Made Ridiculously Simple*, Gladwin, Trattler; MedMaster
13. *Review of Medical Microbiology & Immunology*, Levinson; McGraw-Hill
14. *Illustrated Review: Immunology*, Doan et al.; Lippincott Williams & Wilkins

15. *Illustrated Review: Pharmacology*, Harvey, Champe et al.; Lippincott Williams & Wilkins
16. *Clinical Pharmacology Made Ridiculously Simple*, Olson; MedMaster

17. *Illustrated Review: Biochemistry*, Champe, Harvey et al.; Lippincott Williams & Wilkins
18. *Clinical Biochemistry Made Ridiculously Simple*, Goldberg; MedMaster

19. *Clinical Anatomy Made Ridiculously Simple*, Goldberg; MedMaster
20. *Clinical Neuroanatomy Made Ridiculously Simple*, Goldberg; MedMaster

21. *BRS Physiology (Board Review Series)*, Costanzo, Lippincott Williams & Wilkins
22. *Physiology*, Costanzo; Saunders
23. *Color-Atlas of Physiology*, Silbernagl, Despopoulos; Thieme

24. *BRS Behavioral Science (Board Review Series)*, Fadem; Lippincott Williams & Wilkins

C3 C3 C3 C3 C3 C3 C3 C3 C3 C3 C3 C3 C3 C3 C3 C3

OUTLOOK FOR THE USMLE STEP-2

You will need Chapters 1-3 (Pathology, Microbiology and Pharmacology) for a lightening fast review just prior to taking the USMLE Step-2 exam. My book *USMLE Step-2 Made Ridiculously Simple* will be a big aid for your preparation, but I have not repeated these three chapters in the Step-2 book. It's always best to do your review from books and materials you already have mastered once.

CONTENTS

TABLE OF CONTENTS

PATHOLOGY

A) GENERAL PATHOLOGY

B) ORGAN PATHOLOGY

MICROBIOLOGY

A) GENERAL MICROBIOLOGY

B) BACTERIA

BIOCHEMISTRY

ANATOMY

A) EMBRYOLOGY

B) GROSS ANATOMY

C) NEUROANATOMY

PHYSIOLOGY

SOCIAL SCIENCES

A) PSYCHOLOGY

B) PSYCHOPATHOLOGY

C) STATISTICS

PATHOLOGY

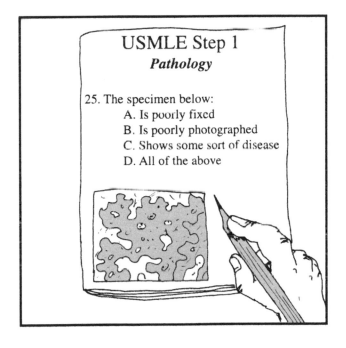

Part A : General Pathology

1.1.) CELL INJURY

A) Reversible Cell Injury:

light microscopy	electron microscopy
- cell swelling - fatty change (liver and heart cells)	- plasma membrane blebbing - mitochondrial swelling

B) Irreversible Cell Injury:

necrosis	apoptosis
- coagulation necrosis - liquefactive necrosis (brain) - caseous necrosis (tuberculosis)	- "programmed cell death"

C) Adaptation to Chronic Injury or Stimuli:

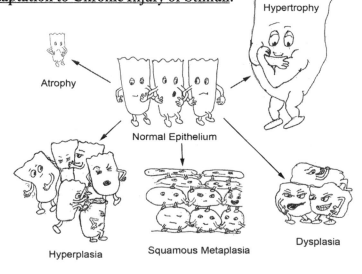

From Zaher: *Pathology Made Ridiculously Simple*, MedMaster, 2007

2

1.2.) WOUND REPAIR

primary intention	secondary intention
- edges are surgically attached - may cause wound contraction	- wound edges are not attached - formation of granulation tissue - takes longer to heal

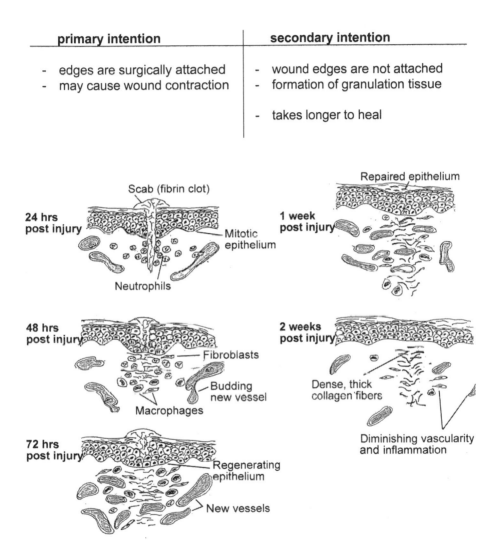

From Zaher: *Pathology Made Ridiculously Simple*, MedMaster, 2007

1.3.) <u>INFLAMMATION</u>

<u>red'n tender – warm'n swollen</u>

Acute inflammation is the response to any kind of damage. It is non-specific, allows immune cells to access the damaged area and clear away dead tissues.

<u>Acute Inflammation</u>:
- increased blood flow
- increased vascular permeability
- emigration of leukocytes

<u>Mediators of Inflammation</u>:

fever	IL-1, prostaglandins
vasodilatation	nitric oxide prostaglandins
exudation	histamine, bradykinin
chemotaxis	complement C5a, IL-8
phagocytosis	complement C3b (opsonin)
pain	prostaglandins, bradykinin

Which parts of the inflammatory response depend on prostaglandins? Can you see how inhibitors of prostaglandin synthesis like aspirin alleviate many symptoms of inflammation (fever, swelling, pain) but not necessarily the inflammatory process itself?

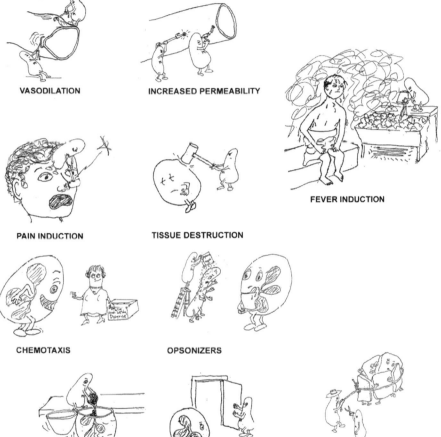

VASODILATION

INCREASED PERMEABILITY

FEVER INDUCTION

PAIN INDUCTION

TISSUE DESTRUCTION

CHEMOTAXIS

OPSONIZERS

PLATELET INDUCTION & INHIBITION

PROMOTION OF WBC PRODUCTION & RELEASE

1.4.) CYTOKINES

> **Overlap and redundancy:**
> - Cytokines have a wide spectrum of effects.
> - Each cytokine may be produced by several cell types.
> - Each leukocyte produces several cytokines.

Main Functions of Cytokines:

during acute inflammation (produced by phagocytes)	IL-1, IL-8, TNF-α
activators of lymphocytes	**T-cells:** IL-1 **B-cells:** IL-2, IL-4, IL-5

Cytokines orchestrate the immune response. It is an almost hopeless task to list all interactions between cells during an inflammatory process. Some of the major ones you may want to know:

antigen presenting cell → IL-1 → activates T lymphocytes (CD4)
(macrophages)

CD4 helper T cell → IL-2 → activates natural killer cells and B cells
               → INF-γ → activates macrophages

T cells → IL-2, 4, 5 → growth and differentiation of
lymphocytes

monocytes → IL-6 → growth and differentiation of
lymphocytes
               → IL-8 → chemotaxis and activation of neutrophils

<u>Major Cytokines:</u>

		PRODUCED BY:	ACTION:
A)	**α-interferon**	leukocytes	- antiviral - induces **MHC-I** expression
	β-interferon	fibroblasts	- antiviral - induces **MHC-I** expression
	γ-interferon	T cells	- activates macrophages - induces **MHC-II** expression *(on macrophages)*
B)	**IL-1**	macrophages	**fever**
	IL-2, IL-3, IL-4, IL-5	T cells	activates many other cells
	IL-6	macrophages fibroblasts	activates many other cells
	IL-7	bone marrow cells	activates many other cells
C)	**TNF-α**	macrophages	like IL-1
D)	**PDGF**	platelets endothelial cells	**proliferation of vascular smooth muscle cells**

Mutation of the IL-2 receptor is the cause of severe combined immune deficiency!

7

1.5.) <u>COMPLEMENT</u>

Complement proteins are enzymes that form a cascade, directed at cleavage of C3. The common final pathway leads to formation of the membrane attack complex. Activation of the alternative pathway does not require specific antibodies (i.e. previous sensitization) but contact with yeast, bacterial cell walls or endotoxins:

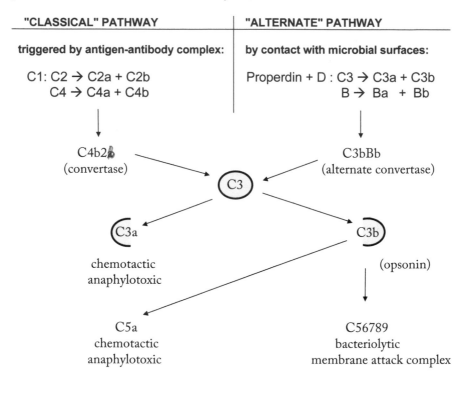

"CLASSICAL" PATHWAY	"ALTERNATE" PATHWAY
triggered by antigen-antibody complex:	**by contact with microbial surfaces:**

$$C1: C2 \rightarrow C2a + C2b$$
$$C4 \rightarrow C4a + C4b$$

$$Properdin + D : C3 \rightarrow C3a + C3b$$
$$B \rightarrow Ba + Bb$$

C4b2b
(convertase)

C3bBb
(alternate convertase)

C3

C3a
chemotactic
anaphylotoxic

C3b
(opsonin)

C5a
chemotactic
anaphylotoxic

C56789
bacteriolytic
membrane attack complex

Complement activity can be measured and is used clinically to follow SLE or immune complex diseases.

1.6.) AUTOANTIBODIES

rheumatoid arthritis	anti-IgG (rheumatoid factor)
systemic lupus	anti-nuclear antibodies (ANA)
drug induced lupus	anti-histone
CREST (Limited scleroderma)	anti-centromere
myasthenia gravis	anti-ACh receptor
Graves' disease	anti-TSH receptor
Hashimoto's thyroiditis	anti-microsomal
Wegener's granulomatosis	anti-neutrophil cytoplasm (ANCA)
primary biliary cirrhosis	anti-mitochondrial
celiac sprue	anti-gliadin
Goodpasture's syndrome	anti glomerular basement membrane

1.7.) WHAT IS AMYLOID?

- *amorphous, eosinophilic <u>extracellular</u> substance*
- *forms aggregates in β-pleated sheets*

- *Congo-Red stain → green birefringence under polarizing microscope*
  (this distinguishes amyloid from other hyaline deposits: collagen, fibrin…)

THE 3 MAIN TYPES OF AMYLOID
AL: Amyloid light chains   ← multiple myeloma
AA: Amyloid associated protein   ← chronic inflammation and aging
Aβ: beta amyloid   ← Alzheimer's disease

1.8.) <u>HYPERSENSITIVITY</u>

	MEDIATORS	SIGNS & SYMPTOMS	EXAMPLES
Type I IgE	- mast cells - basophils → histamine	urticaria erythema bronchioles constrict laryngeal edema shock, death	**anaphylaxis** **asthma** hay fever eczema
Type II IgG, IgM	antibodies bind to cell surface and activate complement	hemolysis	**transfusion reaction** drug reactions erythroblastosis fetalis autoimmune diseases
Type III IgM, IgG	immune complexes get deposited and activate complement	urticaria lymphadenopathy arthritis vasculitis glomerulonephritis	**serum sickness** Arthus reaction SLE
Type IV	T cells (memory cells) activate macrophages and killer cells	erythema with induration	**tuberculin reaction** "delayed hypersensitivity" contact dermatitis multiple sclerosis

Serum sickness: nowadays mostly caused by drugs.
Arthus reaction: edema and necrosis following intradermal injection of drugs.

TRANSPLANT REJECTION
Hyperacute: due to preformed antibodies.
Acute: mostly due to type IV reaction.

1.9.) ONCOGENES

	GENE PRODUCT	DISEASE
c-myc	transcription factor	Burkitt lymphoma
c-abl	tyrosine kinase	CML
bcl-2	inhibits apoptosis	Non-Hodgkin lymphoma
ras	G protein	colon carcinoma

What activates oncogenes?
- Chromosomal rearrangement may bring a dormant oncogene next to some promoter.
- Spontaneous mutations in microRNAs.

1.10.) TUMOR SUPPRESSOR GENES

	DISEASE
RB1	• retinoblastoma osteosarcoma
BRCA-1	• breast cancer • ovarian cancer
p53	• breast carcinoma • colon carcinoma • bronchial carcinomas

HOW ONCOGENES SCREW UP EXPRESSION OF PROTEINS AND REGULATION OF CELL GROWTH:

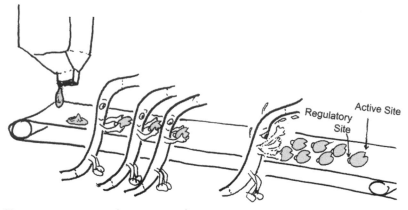

Too many normal gene copies

Regulatory Site

Active Site

Over-stimulated normal gene

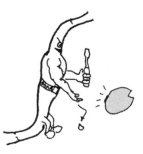

**Mutated gene produces
non-regulated product**

From Zaher: *Pathology Made Ridiculously Simple*, MedMaster, 2007

Tumors sometimes develop several oncogen/suppressor gene abnormalities and become more aggressive.

1.11.) TUMOR MARKERS

Tumor markers are used as follow-up after treatment to detect metastases, but not for screening an asymptomatic population.

CEA	• adenocarcinomas (colon, pancreas, lung)
alpha-fetoprotein	• hepatoma • twin pregnancy • anencephalus
PSA	• prostate carcinoma • more sensitive than acid phosphatase
acid phosphatase	• prostate carcinoma
alkaline phosphatase	• metastases to bones • obstructive biliary disease • Paget's disease

1.12.) METASTASES

Knowing where tumors metastasize to is important: Sometimes you find metastases first and must search for the primary!

	MOST COMMON PRIMARY SITE
brain	lung > breast
bone	breast > lung
liver	colon > stomach > pancreas

1.13.) GENETICS - PEDIGREES

AUTOSOMAL DOMINANT: (vertical pattern)

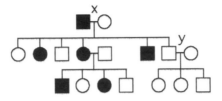

X: Sick person marries healthy person: 50% of children will be sick
males and females have equal risk

Y: Healthy child marries healthy persons: 100% normal offspring

Every sick person has at least one sick parent!

AUTOSOMAL RECESSIVE: (horizontal pattern)

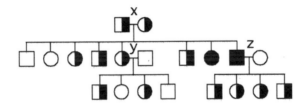

X: If two heterozygotes marry: 25% children will be normal
50% children will be heterozygous
25% children will be sick

Y: Heterozygote marries healthy: 50% children will be normal
50% children will be heterozygous
0% children will be sick

Z: Homozygote marries healthy: 100% children will be heterozygous

X-LINKED RECESSIVE: (oblique pattern)

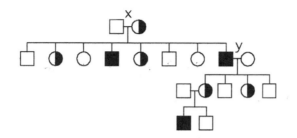

X: Carrier marries healthy male: 50% sons will be sick
    50% sons will be healthy
    100% daughters will be healthy
    50% daughters will be carriers

Y: Sick male marries healthy female: all sons will be healthy
  all daughters will be carriers

Disease tends to skip generations!
Male to male transmission of disease rules out X-linked disease!

☐   healthy male

○   healthy female

■   sick male

●   sick female

◐   heterozygote (carrier)

You should be able to recognize these patterns. Do not memorize the % numbers, try to figure those out by yourself from the chromosomal distributions!

1.14.) AUTOSOMAL RECESSIVE DISEASES

cystic fibrosis	pulmonary infections chronic pancreatitis
phenylketonuria	fair skin, blue eyes mental retardation if untreated
albinism	sunburn, squamous carcinoma of skin
α1-antitrypsin deficiency	emphysema, liver cirrhosis
thalassemias, sickle cell anemias	anemia
glycogen storage diseases	affects liver, muscles, heart (plus hypoglycemia in some)
mucopolysaccharidoses (except Hunter's)	lysosomal storage disease: - facial deformities - mental and physical retardation
sphingolipidoses (except Fabry's)	lysosomal storage disease: - hepatomegaly, splenomegaly
polycystic kidney disease (infant type)	kidney failure
hemochromatosis	liver cirrhosis, diabetes cardiac failure
Chédiak-Higashi syndrome	bacterial and fungal infections of skin and mucous membranes due to impaired leukocyte function

 Albinism: *Melanocytes are present but contain only unpigmented melanosomes.*

1.15.) <u>AUTOSOMAL DOMINANT DISEASES</u>

familial hypercholesterolemia	abnormal LDL receptor coronary artery disease
familial polyposis	colon cancer
spherocytosis	hemolytic anemia
von Willebrand disease	bleeding
Ehlers-Danlos syndrome	stretchy skin sprains, joint dislocations
Marfan syndrome	long bones lens dislocation
achondroplasia	premature ossification dwarfism: short limbs, normal trunk
phacomatoses	benign tumors of eye, skin and brain
Huntington's disease	chorea dementia
polycystic kidney disease (adult type)	kidney failure

 Let's compare the two types of polycystic kidney disease:

ADULT TYPE	INFANT TYPE
• common	• rare
• dominant	• recessive
• berry aneurysms	• liver cysts

1.16.) X-LINKED RECESSIVE DISEASES

hemophilia A and B	bleeding
glucose-6-phosphate deficiency	hemolytic anemia
fragile X	mild mental retardation
Fabry disease	**sphingolipidosis** - cardiomegaly - angiokeratoma
Lesch-Nyhan syndrome	self mutilation + gout
Duchenne	muscle dystrophy - absent dystrophin
Becker	muscle dystrophy - aberrant dystrophin
Bruton's agammaglobulinemia	low or absent B cells
Wiskott-Aldrich syndrome	functional deficiency of B and T cells thrombocytopenia
chronic granulomatous disease	defect of neutrophil free radical formation

Female carriers of X-linked disorders are rarely affected because of the random inactivation of one of the X chromosomes in every cell (Lyon hypothesis).

FRAGILE X CHROMOSOME
Fragile "knob" connected by a stalk to the main part of chromosome X which breaks off easily during karyotyping.
• Female carriers of fragile X may have slight mental retardation.
• Some affected males are mentally normal.

1.17.) TURNER SYNDROME (45, X0)

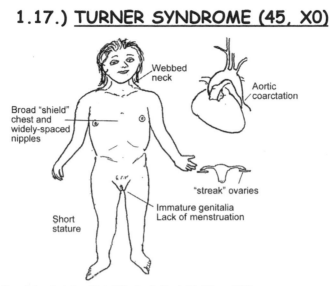

Webbed neck

Aortic coarctation

Broad "shield" chest and widely-spaced nipples

"streak" ovaries

Immature genitalia
Lack of menstruation

Short stature

From Zaher: *Pathology Made Ridiculously Simple*, MedMaster, 2007

1.18.) KLINEFELTER SYNDROME (47, XXY)

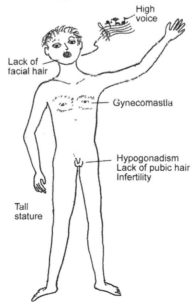

High voice

Lack of facial hair

Gynecomastia

Hypogonadism
Lack of pubic hair
Infertility

Tall stature

From Zaher: *Pathology Made Ridiculously Simple*, MedMaster, 2007

1.19.) DELETIONS

> *Deletion of an entire autosomal chromosome is not compatible with life!*

Partial Deletions:

5p	*cri du chat* syndrome (newborn infants cry like kittens)
11p	congenital absence of iris
13q	retinoblastoma

p: short arm of chromosome

q: long arm of chromosome

A Very Curious Case:

Prader Willi syndrome	**15q11-13 deletion (paternal chromosome)** • severe infantile hypotony • obesity • mental retardation
Angelman syndrome	**15q11-13 deletion (maternal chromosome)** • "happy puppet" syndrome • happy smile, wide-based gait • epilepsy

It's a mystery! Why does a deletion of the maternally versus paternally derived chromosome 15 cause such a different phenotype?

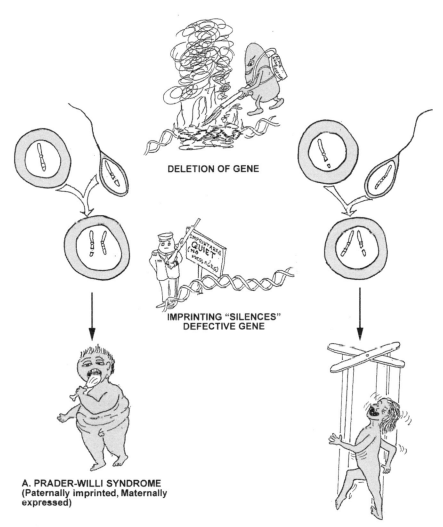

DELETION OF GENE

IMPRINTING "SILENCES"
DEFECTIVE GENE

A. PRADER-WILLI SYNDROME
(Paternally imprinted, Maternally
expressed)

B. ANGELMAN ("HAPPY PUPPET") SYNDROME
(Maternally imprinted, Paternally expressed)

From Zaher: *Pathology Made Ridiculously Simple*, MedMaster, 2007

1.20.) HLA

Major histocompatibility antigens predispose to these diseases:

A3	• hemochromatosis
B27	• ankylosing spondylitis • Reiter's syndrome • ulcerative colitis
DR2	• multiple sclerosis • narcolepsy
DR3	• SLE • IDDM
DR4, Dw4, Dw14	• rheumatoid arthritis • juvenile rheumatoid arthritis

---

RBC antigens are "naturally occurring" antigens:
Patients form antibodies against antigens, which they do not possess.

Leukocyte antigens are not "naturally occurring":
Patients do not form antibodies unless sensitized first (transplants)

MHC Class I	*MHC* Class II
• HLA-A, HLA-B, HLA-C	• HLA-D
• found on all cell surfaces	• found mostly on B-lymphocytes

1.21.) <u>MOST COMMON CAUSES</u>

A) <u>Malignancies</u>:

	INCIDENCE	MORTALITY
men	prostate > lung > colon	lung > prostate > colon
women	breast > lung > colon	lung > breast > colon

 Skin cancers are the most common malignancies, but usually ignored from these statistics because of their low mortality.

> ### <u>Malignancies in Children</u>:
> Most common malignancy **overall**:   leukemia (ALL)
> Most common **solid** malignancy: brain tumors
> Most common solid malignancy **outside CNS**:   neuroblastoma

B) <u>Other Diseases</u>:

acute renal failure	tubular necrosis
nephrotic syndrome	**children:** minimal change glomerulonephritis **adults:** membranous glomerulonephritis
nephritic syndrome	poststreptococcal glomerulonephritis
hypertension	"idiopathic" (= "essential" = we don't know the cause)
anemia	iron deficiency
amenorrhea	pregnancy
chronic pancreatitis	alcoholism
food poisoning	*Clostridia perfringens* *Staph. aureus* toxin

Part B : Organ Pathology

1.22.) SLE

ANA:	sensitive but not specific
anti ds-DNA and anti Sm:	specific but not sensitive

CLINICAL FEATURES OF SLE:

Skin
- Malar rash - spares nasolabial folds
- Photosensitivity

Organs
- Arthritis
- Pleuritis
- Pericarditis
- Renal disease – proteinuria

Blood
- Hemolytic anemia
- Leukopenia
- Lymphocytopenia

Lab
- Antinuclear antibodies
- False positive VDRL (cardiolipin antibodies)
- confirmed by negative FTA-ABS

What is an LE cell ?
Artificially injured leukocytes are mixed with patient's
macrophages. Macrophages then phagocytose nuclei of injured
leukocytes if the patient has SLE.

1.23.) SYSTEMIC SCLEROSIS

excessive fibrosis throughout the body

FEATURES	ANTIBODIES
a) limited = CREST localized scleroderma (fingers, forearm, face)	anti-centromere
b) diffuse systemic widespread scleroderma rapid progression early visceral involvement	anti-Scl 70 (topoisomerase I)

C alcinosis
R aynaud's
E sophageal dysmotility
S clerodactyly
T elangiectasis

1.24.) SJÖGREN'S SYNDROME

immunological destruction of salivary and lacrimal glands

FEATURES	ANTIBODIES
dry eyes, dry mouth	**SS-A** (anti Ro) **SS-B** (anti La)

1.25.) IMMUNODEFICIENCIES

Pay close attention to the clinical features – you can make a diagnostic guess based on the clinical presentation alone:

▼

			CLINICAL FEATURES:
severe combined	lymphopenia (B and T)	X-linked or autosomal	death within first year
DiGeorge's	T cells absent	sporadic	viral infections fungal infections tetany
Bruton's	B cells absent	X-linked	bacterial infections
common variable	B cells present but produce few antibodies	variable	bacterial infections
IgA deficiency	low IgA	autosomal	sinopulmonary infections gastrointestinal infections
Wiskott-Aldrich	low IgM	X-recessive	bacterial infections thrombocytopenia eczema

- most common congenital immunodeficiency: IgA deficiency
- most common acquired immunodeficiency: AIDS

1.26.) BLEEDING DISORDERS

A) The most common <u>inherited</u> bleeding disorder is VonWillebrand's.
B) The most common <u>acquired</u> bleeding disorder is vitamin K deficiency.

		KEY FEATURES
A)	**lack of factor VIII-R** (Von Willebrand disease)	• **aPTT prolonged** • **bleeding time prolonged**
	lack of factor VIII (hemophilia A)	• **aPTT prolonged** • normal bleeding time
	lack of factor IX (hemophilia B)	• **aPTT prolonged** • normal bleeding time
B)	**Vit. K deficiency** (affects factors II, V, VII, IX, X)	• **PT prolonged** • fat malabsorption • antibiotics (diminished gut flora) • coumarin therapy
	ITP (idiopathic thrombocytic purpura)	• immune mediated • children: acute (post viral infection) • adults: often chronic
	TTP (thrombotic thrombocytic purpura)	• young women • microthrombi • fragmented RBCs (helmet cells)

Which disorders result in prolonged bleeding time and which do not? Why?

	depends on:
Bleeding Time:	platelet function
PT:	extrinsic + common pathways
aPTT:	intrinsic + common pathways
TT:	common pathway

27

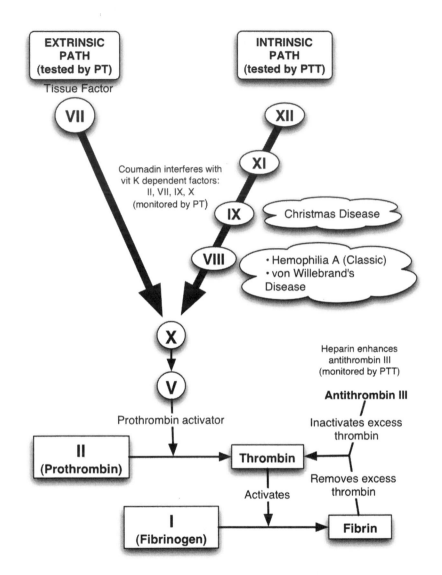

From Zaher: *Pathology Made Ridiculously Simple*, MedMaster, 2007

Measurement of PT has been largely replaced by INR (international normalized ratio), which depends less on the lab standards.

1.27.) HEMOLYTIC ANEMIAS

Anemia results when the bone marrow cannot keep up with the shortened red blood cell survival (normal lifespan of RBC is ~120 days).

A) Hereditary:

	KEY FEATURES
spherocytosis	• autosomal dominant • defective spectrin • splenomegaly
G6PD deficiency	• hemolysis during oxidative stress such as: • viral infections, fava beans, • sulfa drugs, quinine, nitrofurantoin • Heinz bodies (=hemoglobin degradation products)
sickle cell anemia	**HbS ($\alpha_2\beta^s_2$)** • sickling triggered by: hypoxia, dehydration, acidosis • vaso-occlusive crisis • aplastic crisis • sequestration crisis (splenomegaly) • autosplenectomy
α-Thalassemias	**HbH (β_4)** • common in Southeast Asia • hypochromic cells, target cells • Hb Bart (γ_4) $\rightarrow$ hydrops fetalis
β-Thalassemias[1]	**HbA$_2$ ($\alpha_2\delta_2$) and HbF ($\alpha_2\gamma_2$)** • common in Mediterranean and US • hypochromic cells, target cells

[1] ***major*** = *homozygote*, ***minor*** = *heterozygote*

THE ROLE OF SPLEEN

Phagocytes of the spleen remove even slightly abnormal RBCs or RBCs covered with antibodies. However, "therapeutic splenectomy" is NOT beneficial!

B) Immune Mediated:

warm antibodies (usually IgG)	cold antibodies (usually IgM)
active at 37°C	most active at 0~4°C
• drugs • malignancies • SLE	• mycoplasma pneumonia • mononucleosis • lymphoma

Cold antibodies: *Agglutination occurs only in peripheral cool parts of the body → vascular obstruction → Raynaud's phenomenon.*

COOMBS TEST

direct test: detects cell bound antibodies (mix patient's RBCs with anti-IgG)

indirect test: detects free antibodies (mix patient's plasma with normal RBCs)

1.28.) OTHER ANEMIAS

C) Insufficient Production:

	KEY FEATURES

megaloblastic	• hypochromic, macrocytic RBCs
	• hypersegmented neutrophils
	
	• **folate:** anemia
	        no neurological symptoms
	• **B12:** anemia
	        plus neurological symptoms

iron deficiency	• hypochromic, microcytic RBCs • chronic blood loss
aplastic (bone marrow failure)	• viral infections • toxins • drugs : alkylating agents chloramphenicol

In elderly patients with iron deficiency anemia you should always suspect a colorectal malignancy!

Plummer-Vinson:	1. anemia 2. atrophic glossitis 3. esophageal webs

Fanconi Anemia: (autosomal recessive)	1. hypoplastic thumbs 2. absent radii 3. aplastic anemia

(bone marrow DNA is more susceptible to radiation and alkylating agents)

1.29.) RED BLOOD CELLS

If you spot RBCs with "special features" under the microscope, sometimes an instant diagnosis can be made:

Heinz bodies (denatured hemoglobin)	• G6PD deficiency
Howell-Jolly bodies (nuclear fragments)	• post splenectomy
basophil stippling	• lead poisoning
siderocytes	• iron overload • Pappenheimer bodies
reticulocytes (remains of ribosomal RNA)	• increased production/release of RBCs • recovery from hemorrhage

RETICULOCYTE INDEX
Following acute blood loss, the reticulocyte count may double within first 24h. It is important to relate the reticulocyte count to hematocrit in order to correct for the blood loss (so called "reticulocyte index").

RBC SHAPES

RBC INCLUSIONS

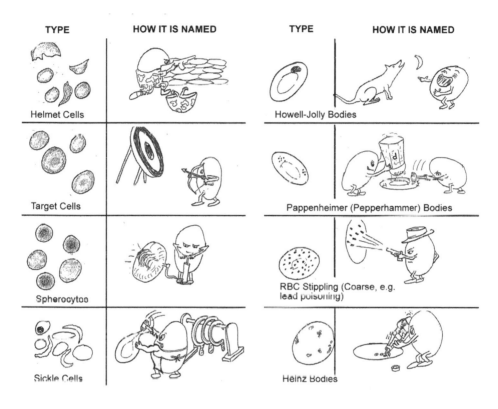

TYPE	HOW IT IS NAMED	TYPE	HOW IT IS NAMED
Helmet Cells		Howell-Jolly Bodies	
Target Cells		Pappenheimer (Pepperhammer) Bodies	
Spherocytes		RBC Stippling (Coarse, e.g. lead poisoning)	
Sickle Cells		Heinz Bodies	

From Zaher: *Pathology Made Ridiculously Simple*, MedMaster, 2007

33

1.30.) NEUTROPENIA

decreased production	• megaloblastic anemia • some leukemias, lymphomas
increased destruction	• immune mediated (Felty's syndrome)
drug induced	• alkylating agents • chloramphenicol • chlorpromazine • sulfonamides • phenylbutazone

1.31.) LEUKOCYTOSIS

neutrophils	• acute infections • stress
eosinophils	• allergy, asthma • parasitic infections
lymphocytes	• tuberculosis • viral infections
monocytes	• tuberculosis • malaria • rickettsia

 Comparing Charts 1.26 and 1.27 – which one is more alarming, leukopenia or leukocytosis?

1.32.) LEUKEMIAS

	ALL	AML	CML	CLL	hairy cell leukemia
	children	any age	young adults	elderly	
	fever petechiae ecchymoses CNS infiltrate	fever petechiae ecchymoses lymphadenopathy (splenomegaly)	fever night sweats splenomegaly	insidious few symptoms low Ig levels infections	hepatomegaly splenomegaly
prognosis : good		depending on type	poor	fair	poor
	lymphoblasts	Auer rods in myeloblasts	Philadelphia chrc.	lymphocytes predominate	pancytopenia TRAP

PHILADELPHIA CHROMOSOME

- if present → better prognosis
- c-abl proto-oncogene on chromosome 9 when translocated to the breakpoint region (bcr) of chromosome 22 forms a fusion gene (bcr/abl).
- This gene encodes a protein with high tyrosine kinase activity.

1.33.) LYMPHOMAS

HODGKIN'S DISEASE	NON-HODGKIN LYMPHOMAS
• spreads in contiguity • no leukemic component • Reed-Sternberg cells	• does not spread in contiguity • often has leukemic component in blood • more common recently !!!

 Reed-Sternberg cells*: Nobody knows where these cells come from! They are binucleated, have prominent nucleoli and clear parachromatin.*

A) SUBTYPES HODGKIN:

	KEY FEATURES
a) lymphocyte predominance b) nodular sclerosis	these have better prognosis
c) mixed cellularity d) lymphocyte depletion	many Reed Sternberg cells → poor prognosis

B) SUBTYPES NON-HODGKIN:

"many subtypes, several classifications, lots of confusion"

CLASS	EXAMPLE
low grade (good prognosis)	small lymphocytic lymphoma
intermediate grade	large cell lymphoma
high grade (poor prognosis)	immunoblastic lymphoma Burkitt lymphoma

---

"Starry sky" pattern of Burkitt lymphoma:
the "stars": benign macrophages
the "sky": matrix of rapidly proliferating neoplastic B cells

---

1.34.) PLASMA CELL NEOPLASIAS

Careful: Myeloma is a plasma cell neoplasm that often presents as a "bone tumor"!

MONOCLONAL GAMMOPATHY	MULTIPLE MYELOMA	WALDENSTRÖM'S
benign	malignant	malignant
usually IgG or IgA	usually IgG or IgA	always IgM
<10% plasma cells in bone marrow	"myeloma cells" (>10% plasma cells infiltrating bone)	"flame cells" (eosinophilic plasma cells)
may convert to multiple myeloma	osteoclast activating factor (→ "punched-out" skull, pelvis, etc.)	hyperviscosity syndrome
	Bence-Jones proteins amyloidosis (tissue deposit of λ-chains)	

M-PROTEIN:
- Monoclonal immunoglobulin secreted by a single clone of aberrant plasma cells.
- May be IgG, IgM etc.

BENCE-JONES PROTEIN:
- Excess light chains (due to unbalanced synthesis of immunoglobulins)
- These are readily filtered through the glomeruli and appear in urine.

1.35.) PHLEBOTHROMBOSIS

Risk factors:	- endothelial injury - slow blood flow - hypercoagulability
Trousseau's sign:	- migratory venous thrombosis - a/w neoplasms

Pulmonary embolism is a major cause of death in the US. Most thrombi originate in the deep veins of the legs and risk factors are the same as for phlebothrombosis.

1.36.) ARTERIOSCLEROSIS

The pathologist distinguishes 4 types of arteriosclerosis depending on location and features:

	KEY FEATURES
atherosclerosis	• large and medium size arteries • fatty streaks • atheromas
Mönckeberg's	• media calcific stenosis • "gooseneck lumps" • small and medium size arteries • asymptomatic
arteriolosclerosis (hyperplastic)	• fibrinoid necrosis • malignant hypertension • "onion skin" hyperplasia
arteriolosclerosis (hyaline)	• diabetes mellitus • thickened basement membrane

Pathogenesis of Arteriosclerosis:

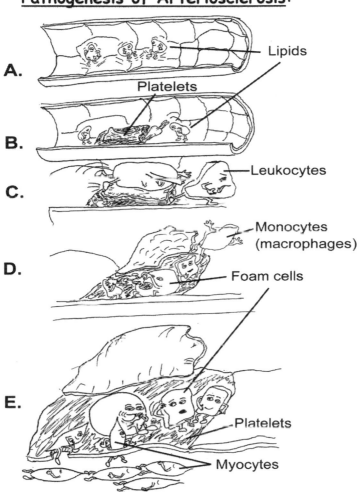

From Zaher: *Pathology Made Ridiculously Simple*, MedMaster, 2007

A) Injury of the vascular endothelium.

B) Lipids and platelets adhere to damaged surface.

C) Leukocytes and platelets release growth factors → smooth muscle proliferation.

D) Macrophages become foam cells.

E) Foam cells aggregate to "fatty streaks", the beginning formation of an atherosclerotic plaque.

1.37.) ARTERITIS

Try to memorize which vessels are affected by which diseases:

	KEY FEATURES
hypersensitivity arteritis	• small vessels • lesions all at same stage • cryoglobulins • a/w Henoch-Schönlein purpura
polyarteritis nodosa	• small and medium vessels • kidneys, heart, muscles, skin • can be fatal but responds well to steroids
thromboangiitis obliterans (Buerger's)	• small and medium vessels • in smokers
giant cell arteritis	**temporal artery** • sudden blindness • female > male • a/w polymyalgia rheumatica
Wegener's	• upper respiratory vasculitis • lower respiratory vasculitis • glomerulonephritis
Takayasu	**= pulseless disease"** • aorta / large arteries • Asian females
Kawasaki	**= mucocutaneous lymph node syndrome** • coronary artery aneurysms • fever, conjunctivitis, maculopapular rash • Japanese children

Giant cell arteritis: *Early diagnosis is essential to prevent permanent loss of vision!*

1.38.) ANEURYSMS

	KEY FEATURES
atherosclerotic	• fusiform • abdominal aorta • hypertension
syphilitic	• saccular • ascending aorta • a/w aortic insufficiency
dissecting (not a "true" aneurysm)	• aorta (ascending or descending) • hypertension • Marfan syndrome
berry	• congenital • circle of Willis • a/w polycystic kidney disease (adult form)
micro	• cerebral : hypertension • retinal : diabetes

Abdominal aortic aneurysms are the most common form because of atherosclerosis and hypertension. Rupture has very high mortality.

You should know which aneurysms are typical for each location.

1.39.) HEART SOUNDS

	OCCURS IN:	SOUNDS LIKE:
mitral valve prolapse	• young women • Marfan syndrome	• midsystolic click
mitral stenosis	• rheumatic heart disease • atrial fibrillation	• diastolic rumble
mitral regurgitation	• MI (papillary muscle) • acute rheumatic fever • endocarditis	• holosystolic murmur • transmitted *to axilla*
aortic stenosis	• congenital • degenerative calcifications	• systolic murmur • transmitted *to carotid artery*
aortic regurgitation	• "water hammer" pulse	• diastolic murmur • "pistol shots" in femoral art.
patent ductus arteriosus	• kept open by PGE_2, PGI_2	• continuous murmur ("machine like")

Pulsus parvus et tardus = *"small and weak"* → *aortic stenosis*

1.40.) CONGENITAL HEART DEFECTS

R→L shunts (deoxygenated blood gets into the systemic circulation) are more serious than L→R shunts (systemic blood gets into pulmonary circulation).

A) Types

ACYANOTIC (L→R)	CYANOTIC (R→L)	OBSTRUCTIVE

• VSD [1]
• ASD
  ostium primum
  ostium secundum
 	
• PDA
	• Fallot's tetralogy [1]
	• transposition of great vessels
	• persistent truncus arteriosus
	  Eisenmenger : reversal of
	  L→R shunt due to pulmonary
	  hypertension
		• coarctation of aorta
		  infants: preductal
		  adults: postductal
		
		• pulmonary or aortic
		  stenosis or atresia

[1] *most common cyanotic and acyanotic defects respectively*

B) Heart Defects are common in many syndromes:

	CARDIAC DEFECT PLUS:
fetal alcohol syndrome	• microcephaly • short, upturned nose, long philtrum
fetal hydantoin syndrome	• microcephaly • nail hypoplasia
isotretinoin (Vit. A)	• hydrocephalus • cleft palate
TORCH (intrauterine infection)	• microcephaly • auditory and visual defects
syphilis	• bullous skin lesions (palms, soles) • Hutchinson's teeth • saber shins

> **TORCH:** Toxoplasmosis, Rubella, CMV, Herpes

C) Transposition of Great Arteries

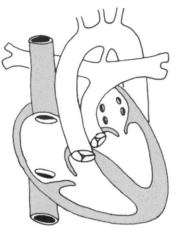

From Goldberg: *Clinical Anatomy Made Ridiculously Simple*, MedMaster, 2007

D) Tetralogy of Fallot

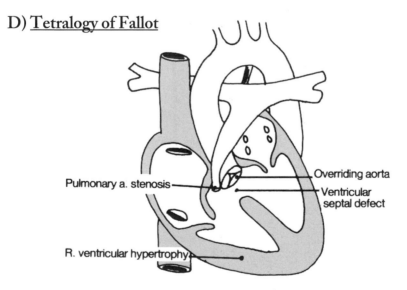

From Goldberg: *Clinical Anatomy Made Ridiculously Simple*, MedMaster, 2007

1.41.) ISCHEMIC HEART DISEASE

	SIGNS & TREATMENT
stable angina	• exercise • ST depression • relieved by rest ➤ *TX : nitroglycerin*
unstable angina	• at rest or crescendo like • often leads to MI ➤ *unresponsive to nitroglycerin*
Prinzmetal's angina	• at rest • ST elevated ➤ *TX : Ca^{2+} antagonists*

myocardial infarction	• during exercise or REM sleep
	• ST elevation
	• T inversion
	
	➤ *TX : nitroglycerin*
	     morphine
	     lidocaine

You should be able to make a diagnostic guess based on the clinical presentation. A suspect MI needs to be confirmed by ECG and enzymes:

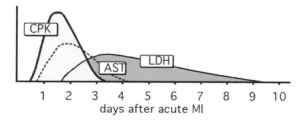

days after acute MI

1.42.) MYOCARDIAL INFARCTION

Which complications occur early, which ones occur late?
How long does it take for an MI to heal?

TIME AFTER MI	GROSS CHANGE	MICROSCOPIC CHANGE
30 minutes	-	mitochondrial swelling
4-12 h	-	edema, hemorrhage
18-24 h	pallor	neutrophilic infiltrate
24-72 h	pallor	coagulation necrosis loss of nuclei heavy neutrophil. Infiltrate
3-7 days	central softening hyperemic borders	resorption of dead myofibers
10 days	max. soft and yellow hyperemic borders	granulation tissue
8 weeks	gray and firm scar	scar

Complications:

Arrhythmia: most common cause of death in first hours after MI
Myocardial rupture: highest risk 1~2 weeks after MI

most common

least common

Arrhythmia
Congestive heart failure
Cardiogenic shock
Muscle rupture

1.43.) HEART FAILURE

Left and right heart failure have very different signs and symptoms. It is important that you recognize the clinical presentation:

LEFT	RIGHT
CAUSES: • ischemic heart disease • arterial hypertension • valvular disease	• left sided heart failure • lung disease • primary pulmonary hypertension

CONSEQUENCES:
 	
• pulmonary congestion
  → dyspnea, orthopnea
 	
• renal hypoperfusion
  → salt retention
	• increased venous pressure
	  › edema
	  → liver congestion ("nutmeg liver")
	  → ascites

1.44.) ENDOCARDITIS

A) INFECTIVE   B) NON-INFECTIVE

ACUTE	SUBACUTE	MARANTIC	LIBMAN SACKS
• **Staph. aureus** • **Streptococci**	• **Strep. viridans** • **gram negative bacilli**	• a/w chronic illnesses	• SLE
• previously normal valves	• previously abnormal valves	• thrombotic (platelet and fibrin deposits)	• verrucous lesions on both sides of valve leaflets
• Janeway lesions	• Roth spots • Osler nodes		
• high fever, chills • hematuria	• low grade fever		

More common on the USMLE than in real life:

Janeway lesions:	non-tender, macular patches on palms and soles (septic emboli).
Roth spots:	oval retinal hemorrhages with pale center.
Osler nodes:	red, tender lesions on finger and toe pulps.

1.45.) PERICARDITIS

The space between the visceral and parietal pericardium normally contains ~20mL of clear fluid. The pathologist distinguishes 3 types of pericarditis based on the appearance of this fluid:

	KEY FEATURES
fibrinous	• transmural myocardial infarction, • Dressler syndrome • "bread and butter" appearance
serous	• viral infections (often Coxsackie) • uremia
suppurative	• bacterial infections • fungal infections • parasitic infections

CLINICAL SIGNS
➤ low-grade fever
➤ pericardial friction rub: chest pain, aggravated by movement of trunk
➤ pulsus paradoxus: nothing paradox about it: just a normal inspiratory fall in blood pressure that is exaggerated

Dressler syndrome: *Delayed pericarditis (2-10 weeks after infarction) due to autoantibodies. Responds well to corticosteroids.*

1.46.) <u>RHEUMATIC FEVER</u>

Rheumatic fever occurs mostly in school-age children with untreated streptococcal pharyngitis.

ACUTE RHEUMATIC FEVER	RHEUMATIC HEART DISEASE
occurs 1-4 weeks after tonsillitis group A β-hemolytic streptococci	occurs many years after rheumatic fever often asymptomatic
common in children 5-15 years	fibrotic, deformed, calcified lines of closure on valve leaflets
Major Jones Criteria • polyarthritis • erythema • subcutaneous nodules • chorea • carditis	**mitral valve** > aortic valve

Carditis of rheumatic fever:
pericarditis → serous effusions
myocarditis → heart failure
endocarditis → valvular damage

ASCHOFF BODY (= Granuloma)
- focal interstitial myocardial inflammation
- enlarged macrophages (Anitschkow cells)

Most common clinical presentation is migratory polyarthritis, lasting 2-3 weeks, accompanied by fever.

1.47.) OBSTRUCTIVE LUNG DISEASES

Reduced airflow either because airway resistance is high or because elastic recoil of lungs is low → **FRC and TLC are high.**

	KEY FEATURES
emphysema	• pink puffers , barrel chest • panacinar • (α1-antitrypsin deficiency, lower lobes) • centrilobular • (smoking, upper lobes)
chronic bronchitis	• blue bloaters • chronic irritation / infections • hypertrophy of submucosal glands
asthma	• expiratory wheezing • extrinsic (triggered by allergens) • intrinsic (triggered by cold, exercise) [1] • aspirin induced
bronchiectasis	• result of chronic infections • Kartagener's : immotile cilia

[1] *intrinsic asthma is a common problem of ice skaters.*

<u>COPD:</u> usually coexisting:

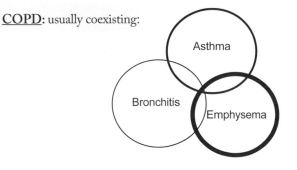

The REID Index = Glands (B) / Wall (A)

The REID index is the ratio between the thickness of submucosal mucus secreting glands and the wall thickness between epithelium and cartilage of the bronchi. It is used for research and autopsy only, not for diagnosis.

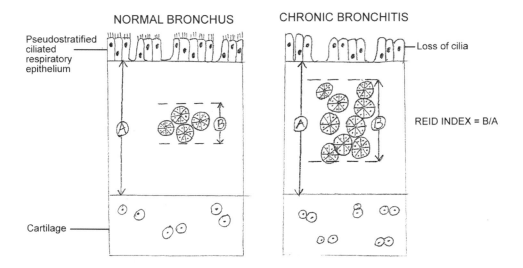

From Zaher: *Pathology Made Ridiculously Simple*, MedMaster, 2007

1.48.) <u>RESTRICTIVE LUNG DISEASES</u>

Elastic recoil of lungs is large → FRC , VC and TLC are low.

	KEY FEATURES
adult ARDS	• acute diffuse alveolar damage • (causes: sepsis, shock, pancreatitis, toxins)
neonatal ARDS	• insufficient lecithin synthesis by type 2 pneumocytes
pneumoconiosis	• coal : "tattooing", black sputum • anthracosis : carbon dust • asbestosis : fibrous silicates, dry cough • berylliosis : **Type IV hypersensitivity**
hypersensitivity pneumonitis	• acute : **(Type III)** fever, cough, dyspnea, leukocytosis • chronic : **(Type IV)** peribronchial granulomas • Farmer's lung, pigeon breeder's lung etc.
Goodpasture syndrome	• **(Type II)**, antibodies against basal membrane • hemoptysis, rapidly progressive glomerulonephritis
pulmonary hemosiderosis	• like Goodpasture's but without renal involvement
alveolar proteinosis	• overproduction of surfactant like material
eosinophilic pneumonia	• acute (Löffler's) : **Type I hypersensitivity** • chronic
diffuse idiopathic fibrosis	• interstitial pneumonitis and fibrosis • hyperplasia of type II pneumocytes
collagen vascular disorders	• scleroderma, SLE, Wegener's, RA etc.

Please review the immunological mechanisms of hypersensitivity (chart 1.6) involved in restrictive lung diseases.

PULMONARY EDEMA AND IT'S CAUSES:

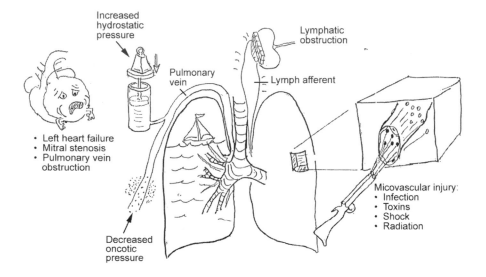

Increased hydrostatic pressure

Lymphatic obstruction

Pulmonary vein

Lymph afferent

- Left heart failure
- Mitral stenosis
- Pulmonary vein obstruction

Micovascular injury:
- Infection
- Toxins
- Shock
- Radiation

Decreased oncotic pressure

From Zaher: *Pathology Made Ridiculously Simple*, MedMaster, 2007

*Edema occurs whenever **filtration > resorption + lymph flow***
The driving force for filtration and resorption is determined by the differences in hydrostatic pressures and oncotic pressures.

1.49.) PNEUMONIA

Sudden fever, cough, sputum and dyspnea are the signs of "classic pneumonia". It is a lobar pneumonia (affecting entire lobe of lung) caused by *Pneumococcus*.

	CAUSED BY
bronchopneumonia	• *Haemophilus* • *Pseudomonas*
lobar pneumonia ("classic")	• *Pneumococcus* • *Klebsiella*
atypical pneumonia [1]	• viral • *Mycoplasma*
Legionnaire's disease [2] (severe lobar pneumonia)	• *Legionella*

[1] *most frequent in young adults (college students)*

[2] *more frequent in elderly, via water reservoirs*
no person to person transmission

What is atypical about "atypical pneumonia"?
- more gradual onset
- dry, non productive cough
- minimal signs of pulmonary involvement during physical examination
- prominent extrapulmonary symptoms, myalgia etc.
- prominent chest x-ray ("looks worse than patient")

1.50.) LUNG TUMORS

A) NOT SMOKING RELATED:

benign	• adenoma • leiomyoma • hamartoma
carcinoid	• potentially malignant • carcinoid <u>syndrome</u> suggests widespread metastasis
adeno CA	• peripheral, weakly related to smoking

B) SMOKING RELATED:

squamous CA	• central, strong correlation with smoking • paraneoplastic: **PTH**-like peptide
small cell CA	• central, hormone producing, aggressive • paraneoplastic: **ACTH, ADH**
large cell CA	• peripheral, poorly differentiated adeno or squamous CA

<u>Clinical features:</u> (overall less than 5% 10-year survival)

- Pancoast tumor (apex of lung)   → compressing cervical sympathetic chain
                                                  → Horner's syndrome)

- Compression of recurrent laryngeal nerve → hoarseness
- Obstruction of superior vena cava → facial swelling

1.51.) <u>GLOMERULONEPHRITIS - I</u>

Clinically you must distinguish between nephritic and nephrotic syndrome:

NEPHRITIC SYNDROME	NEPHROTIC SYNDROME
• hematuria • RBC casts	• severe proteinuria • hypoalbuminemia • hyperlipidemia • edema
• post streptococcal GN	• adults: membranous GN • children: minimal change GN

The underlying pathology is established by renal biopsy and determines treatment and prognosis. But be aware that pathological changes and clinical manifestations often vary over time. You need to know which ones have a good and which have a poor prognosis:

diffuse proliferative GN	• poststreptococcal GN • good prognosis
mesangiocapillary GN (membranoproliferative GN)	• young adults, idiopathic • poor prognosis
focal-segmental GN	• aggressive variant of minimal change GN
Goodpasture's (anti-GBM antibodies)	• young males • pulmonary hemorrhage
Berger's (IgA nephropathy)	• very common, lasts 1-2 days • mild proteinuria, hematuria in children • follows respiratory infection

1.52.) GLOMERULONEPHRITIS - II

A) GOOD PROGNOSIS:

	CLINICAL FEATURES	PATHOLOGIC FEATURES
minimal change (lipoid nephrosis)	- most common nephrotic syndrome in children - insidious onset	- no immune complexes - **loss of foot processes**
diffuse proliferative	- nephritic/nephrotic - post streptococcal, SLE	- proliferation of mesangium and epithelium - **subepithelial deposits**

B) POOR PROGNOSIS:

	CLINICAL FEATURES	PATHOLOGIC FEATURES
membranous	- most common nephrotic syndrome in young adults - insidious onset	- thickening of GBM - **subepithelial deposits** of immune complexes - 85% unknown antigen
membrano- proliferative	- variable presentation	- GBM thickening plus proliferation of mesangium - **subendothelial or intra-membranous** deposits of immune complexes - "tram track" appearance
focal segmental	- related to minimal change?	- segmental sclerosis - usually IgM deposits (**IgA in Berger's**)
rapidly progressive	- aggressive variant of any other type	- **crescents** - oliguria, uremia

1.53.) UROLITHIASIS

Kidney stones form when the urine is supersaturated with salts. You need to know which salts precipitate in alkaline and which ones precipitate in acidic urine:

calcium	• 80% of cases • precipitates in **alkaline** urine ➤ *TX : thiazide* *potassium phosphate*
Mg - NH$_3$ – Phosphate "triple stones"	• (staghorn calculi) • urinary tract infections (*Proteus*) • precipitates in **alkaline** urine ➤ *TX : antibiotics* *acidification*
uric acid	• gout • leukemia • precipitates in **acidic** urine ➤ *TX : bicarbonate*
cystine	• congenital defect in dibasic • amino acid transporter • precipitates in **acidic** urine ➤ *TX : bicarbonate*

 Renal colic: *excruciating, intermittent pain, radiating from flank area across abdomen to genital region.*

1.54.) VENEREAL DISEASES

	CAUSED BY: ▼	CLINICAL FEATURES	TREATMENT
gonorrhea	Neisseria gonorrhoeae	purulent urethritis	ceftriaxone
trichomoniasis	Trichomonas vaginalis	men: asymptomatic or NGU female: vaginitis	metronidazole
non-gonococcal urethritis	Chlamydia trachomatis [1]	urethritis, PID	doxycycline
lymphogranuloma venereum	Chlamydia trachomatis [1]	ulcer (**painless**) lymphadenopathy	doxycycline
granuloma inguinale	C. donovani	multiple ulcerating papules lymph nodes not involved [2]	tetracycline
chancroid	Hemophilus ducreyi	soft chancre (**painful**)	ceftriaxone
syphilis (I) **syphilis (II)** **syphilis (III)**	Treponema pallidum	hard chancre (**painless**) cond. lata (flat brown papules) gumma	penicillin G
condyloma acuminatum	HPV	"red warts"	cryotherapy
genital herpes	HSV2 or HSV1	recurrent vesicles (**painful**)	acyclovir

[1] different strains   [2] induration is of subcutaneous tissue

Yeast infection (*Candida*) is not sexually transmitted, i.e. not a STD

1.55.) <u>TESTICULAR TUMORS</u>

Patients present with a scrotal mass and you need to examine these carefully:
Testicular masses usually are malignant while extra-testicular ones often are
benign. Prognosis depends on tumor size and histology:

A) <u>Germ Cell Tumors</u> (common):

	KEY FEATURES
seminoma	• uniform polyhedral • radiosensitive, good prognosis
embryonal	• more aggressive • hemorrhage, necrosis
choriocarcinoma	• highly malignant • gynecomastia
yolk sac	• most common in children • serum AFP ↑ • very aggressive
teratoma	• contains multiple tissue types • often malignant!

B) <u>Non Germ Cell Tumors</u> (rare):

Leydig cell	• androgens, estrogens, corticosteroids • usually benign
Sertoli cell	• little or no hormone production
lymphoma	• mostly in elderly

1.56.) OVARIAN TUMORS

A) Surface Epithelium (most common):

	KEY FEATURES
serous	• cysts, ciliated epithelium
mucinous	• cysts, non ciliated epithelium
endometrioid	• glandular tissue
clear cell	• rare, malignant
Brenner	• rare, benign • nests of <u>transitional</u> epithelium in stroma

B) Germ Cell Tumors (less common):

teratoma	• usually mature (benign) [1]
dysgerminoma	• like seminoma, radiosensitive
endodermal sinus tumor	• like yolk sac tumor, AFP ↑
choriocarcinoma	• produces HCG

[1] *also called dermoid cyst*

C) Sex Cord Stroma Cell Tumors (rare):

granulosa-theca	• estrogens and androgens
Sertoli-Leydig	• androgens → masculinization
fibroma	• Meig's syndrome → ascites

Compare ovarian tumors side by side with testicular tumors. Which correspond to which?

1.57.) ENDOMETRIUM

Proliferation of endometrial glands due to estrogen stimulation results in:

POLYPS	HYPERPLASIA	CARCINOMA
• excessive bleeding • rarely malignant transformation	• excessive bleeding • premalignant	• usually adenocarcinoma • may be asymptomatic or present with bleeding **risk factors** age >40 years early menarche late menopause nulliparity obesity

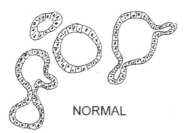

NORMAL

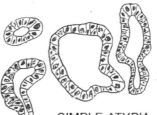

SIMPLE ATYPIA

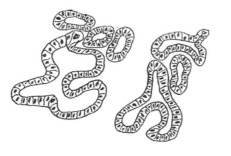

COMPLEX ATYPIA

SEVERE ATYPIA

From Zaher: *Pathology Made Ridiculously Simple*, MedMaster, 2007

1.58.) PLACENTA

HYDATIDIFORM MOLE (80% benign)	CHORIOCARCINOMA (malignant)

• older pregnant woman
• uterus larger than expected
• grape-like cystic material
 	
• HCG elevated
	• derived from: hydatidiform mole (50%)
	                    pregnancy (25%)
	                    abortion (25%)
	
	• HCG elevated

 Moles are due to fertilization of ovum by multiple sperms:

Complete hydatidiform mole:
o no embryo or placenta
o 46,XX of exclusively paternal origin

Partial hydatidiform mole:
o embryo and placenta are present
o triploid or tetraploid karyotype

1.59.) BREAST

NORMAL DUCT

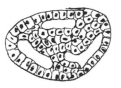

DUCTAL HYPERPLASIA

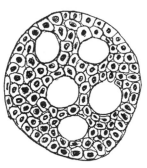

ATYPICAL DUCTAL HYPERPLASIA
(Continuum to ductal carcinoma-in-situ)

From Zaher: *Pathology Made Ridiculously Simple*, MedMaster, 2007

<u>Most breast masses are benign. Please compare carefully:</u>

FIBROCYSTIC CHANGE	BREAST CANCER
• often bilateral • multiple nodules • menstrual variation • may regress during pregnancy	• often unilateral • single mass • no cyclic variations

<u>BENIGN TUMORS</u>

fibroadenoma	• single, movable nodule
cystosarcoma phyllodes	• rapidly growing, may become huge
intraductal papilloma	• nipple discharge (bloody or serous) • nipple retraction

<u>MALIGNANT TUMORS</u>

ductal carcinoma	• most common
lobular carcinoma	• if receptor positive → better prognosis
Paget's disease of nipple	• older woman • poor prognosis

> **<u>Risk factors for breast cancer:</u>**
> same as for endometrial cancer (1.57)

 5% of women with breast cancer carry BRCA1 or BRCA2 genes. Women without positive family history probably do not carry these genes and screening for BRCA1 or BRCA2 is not recommended.

1.60.) MOUTH

Some diseases cause characteristic changes of the lips, gums or tongue:

bleeding gums	Vit. C deficiency
glossitis, cheilosis	Vit. B2 deficiency
smooth beefy red tongue	Vit. B12 deficiency
strawberry tongue	scarlet fever
Koplik's spots (white dots on red background)	measles
thrush (white, removable)	Candida albicans

1.61.) DIVERTICULAS & HERNIAS

A) Esophageal Diverticula:

PULSION DIVERTICULA (Zenker's)	TRACTION DIVERTICULA
• "false" (mucosa only)	• "true" (all layers)
• at junction of pharynx/esophagus	• mid part of esophagus
• dysphagia, regurgitation	• asymptomatic

 Compare the anatomic features of the two types of diverticula and review the layers of the gastrointestinal tube: mucosa → lamina propria → muscularis mucosa → submucosa → circular muscle layer → longitudinal muscle layer.

B) Hiatal Hernias:

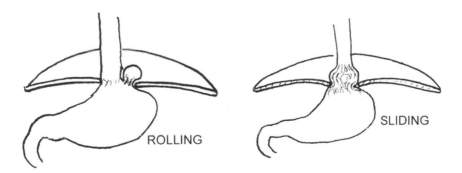

ROLLING

SLIDING

From Zaher: *Pathology Made Ridiculously Simple*, MedMaster, 2007

1.62.) GASTRITIS

"Gastritis" is 4 different, unrelated diseases:

ACUTE EROSIVE	CHRONIC TYPE A	CHRONIC TYPE B	MÉNÉTRIER'S
focal damage • alcohol • NSAIDs • stress	fundal gastritis • autoimmune • pernicious anemia • achlorhydria	antral gastritis • *H. pylori*	thickened mucosa

Patients on intensive care often develop acute erosive gastritis. You may want to give prophylactic proton-pump inhibitor.

H. pylori is associated with:
- chronic gastritis type B
- gastric and duodenal peptic ulcers
- carcinoma of stomach

1.63.) GASTROENTERITIS

TOXIN INGESTION	BACTERIA	NON-BACTERIAL
Staph. aureus *Cl. botulinum*	**toxigenic** *Campylobacter* [1] *E. coli* *Salmonella* **invasive** *Shigella*	Rotavirus (children) Parvovirus (adults) *Candida* *Entameba histolytica* *Giardia lamblia*

[1] *very common cause of bacterial gastroenteritis in US !*

1.64.) POLYPOSIS OF COLON

Step by Step:

Absence of APC (a tumor suppressor gene) causes familial adenomatous polyposis. If the adenoma cells develop additional mutations of the normal gene on the other allele, they will become cancerous!

		POLYPS PLUS: ◀	CANCER RISK:
familial adenomatous polyposis	autosomal dominant	(none)	almost 100%
Gardner's	autosomal dominant	+ skin and bone tumors	almost 100%
Turcot's	autosomal recessive	+ brain tumors	high
Peutz-Jeghers	autosomal dominant	+ melanin pigmentation of lips, palms and soles	very low

Follow-up and genetic counseling:

- Patient's offspring has 50% risk of disease.
- Screen annually until age 35 (flexible sigmoidoscopy)
- If polyps develop → need to remove colon

1.65.) INFLAMMATORY BOWEL DISEASE

A favorite on the USMLE. You must memorize the differences:

CROHN'S DISEASE	ULCERATIVE COLITIS
• rectum often spared • ileum often involved	• begins at rectum and progresses • towards ileocecal junction
• skip lesions • transmural	• continuous • mucosa / submucosa only
• granulomas • strictures and fissures	• crypt abscesses • pseudopolyps
• more pain, less bleeding	• more bleeding, less pain
	complications: - increased risk of colon carcinoma - toxic megacolon

1.66.) MALABSORPTION

celiac sprue	• toxic/allergic reaction against gluten • flat mucosal surface • avoid wheat • rice and corn are O.K.
tropical sprue	• cause unknown
Whipple's disease	• malabsorption + anemia + arthritis • *Tropheryma whippelii* • PAS positive macrophages found in mucosa ➤ *TX : penicillin or tetracycline*

Symptoms are due to (1.) osmotically active substances remaining in the GI tract (diarrhea, bloating) and (2.) nutritional deficiencies (weight loss, glossitis, megaloblastic anemia).

A) <u>Ulcerative Colitis</u>:

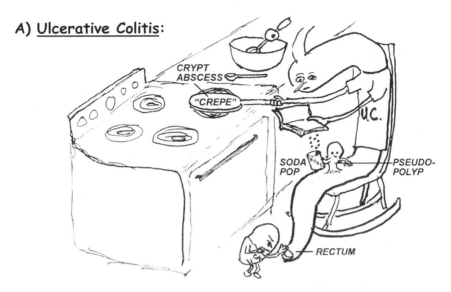

From Zaher: *Pathology Made Ridiculously Simple*, MedMaster, 2007

B) <u>Crohn's Disease</u>:

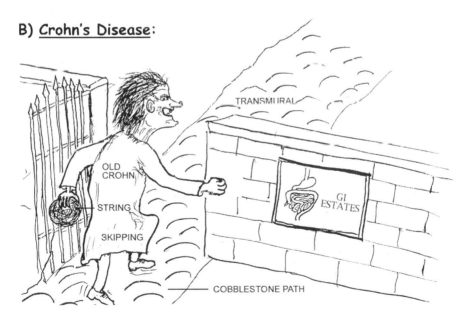

From Zaher: *Pathology Made Ridiculously Simple*, MedMaster, 2007

1.67.) <u>CHOLELITHIASIS</u>

Cholesterol is insoluble in water and must be incorporated in salt-phospholipid micelles in the bile. Supersaturation results in crystal formation and stones.

<u>STONE TYPES</u>:

CHOLESTEROL	MIXED	PIGMENT (BILIRUBIN)
• radiolucent [1] • often a single stone • Westerners • **fat, female, forty, fertile**	• most common • 15% radiopaque	• radiolucent [1] • a/w hemolytic anemia • Asians

[1] *not detectable on plain radiograph*

Porcelain Gallbladder: - calcium deposits in wall
                                    - high risk of malignancy

Strawberry Gallbladder: - asymptomatic lipid deposits
                                    - not related to cholelithiasis
                                    - no cancer risk

Charcot's triad = signs of cholangitis:
1. acute onset fever, sepsis
2. RUQ pain
3. jaundice

1.68.) <u>CARCINOMAS</u>

Curiously, gallbladder and bile duct carcinomas are quite different:

GALLBLADDER CA	BILE DUCT CA
• female • cholelithiasis • porcelain gallbladder	• male • chronic infections • liver fluke (*Clonorchis sinensis*)

1.69.) JAUNDICE

occurs if serum bilirubin > 2 mg/dl
direct = conjugated   = water soluble
indirect = unconjugated = insoluble (bound to albumin)

	DUE TO:	SERUM BILIRUBIN
prehepatic	hemolysis	unconjugated
hepatic	hepatitis	conjugated and unconjugated
posthepatic	cholestasis	conjugated

CONGENITAL CAUSES OF JAUNDICE :

Gilbert	auto-dominant	impaired uptake (mild)
Crigler-Najjar	auto-dominant or auto-recessive	impaired uptake (very severe)
Rotor	auto-recessive	impaired hepatocellular secretion

Physiologic jaundice of the newborn:
- *2-3 days after birth*
- *lasts less than 1 week*
- *more severe in prematures*
  (immature liver enzymes abd immature blood-brain barrier)

1.70.) HEPATITIS

The clinical presentation varies from minor flu-like illness to fulminant, fatal liver failure. Histopathology is similar, regardless of virus. You should know serum markers (for diagnosis) and routes of transmission (for prevention):

A	RNA	• viruses in feces • acute : IgM • late : IgG	• **fecal/oral** • 2-6 weeks [2] • 0% chronic
B	**DNA**	• HBs-Ag , earliest marker [1] • HBe-Ag, infective state	• **parenteral** • 2-6 months [2] • 10% chronic
C	RNA	• antibody ELISA	• **parenteral** • 1-2 months [2] • 50% chronic
Delta	RNA	• incomplete RNA • requires Hep B virus for replication	• **parenteral**
E	RNA		• **fecal oral** • SE Asia • often fulminant in pregnant woman

[1] *also indicates carrier state*   [2] *incubation times*

CHRONIC HEPATITIS (> 6 months):

chronic persistent hepatitis
• inflammation limited to portal triad

chronic active hepatitis
• inflammation beyond portal triad
   (piece meal necrosis)

1.71.) HEPATITIS B SEROLOGY

These markers are important for diagnosis and follow-up:

HBeAg	• appears after HBsAg • disappears before HBsAg • indicates infectivity!
HBsAg	• appears before onset of symptoms • persists for 3-4 months • if > 6 months: chronic carrier state
anti-HBsAg	• appears a few weeks after HBsAg has disappeared • indicates recovery and immunity
anti HBcAg	• only marker present during "window period"

"Window period": time after HBsAg disappears but before anti-HBsAg appears in patient's serum.

1.72.) TOXIC HEPATITIS

Several drugs may cause hepatitis in a predictable, dose-depend manner. A few drugs elicit a severe, idiosyncratic (=dose-independent) hepatitis in susceptible patients:

PREDICTABLE	IDIOSYNCRATIC
➤ acetaminophen ➤ amanita ➤ carbon tetrachloride ➤ methotrexate	➤ halothane ➤ isoniazid ➤ methyl-DOPA

1.73.) CIRRHOSIS

A) Most common types of cirrhosis:

ALCOHOL (60%)	TOXINS, VIRAL (30%)	BILIARY (10%)
early: micronodular **late:** macronodular	macronodular	micronodular
Mallory bodies[1] in <u>acute</u> hepatitis !		autoimmune disease anti-mitochondrial antibodies

[1] *swollen hepatocytes that contain cytoplasmic inclusions of a fibrillar protein. Common in, but NOT specific, for alcohol hepatitis!*

B) Rare types of cirrhosis:

HEMOCHROMATOSIS: - accumulation of hemosiderin
triad of (1.) cirrhosis, (2.) diabetes mellitus and (3.) skin pigmentation

WILSON'S DISEASE: - accumulation of copper
- decreased serum ceruloplasmin

1.74.) LIVER CARCINOMA

METASTATIC	HEPATOCELLULAR	CHOLANGIOCARCINOMA
most common	90% of <u>primary</u> ones	10% of <u>primary</u> ones
• from breast • from lung • from colon	HBV and HCV aflatoxin AFP ↑	more common in Asia (due to liver flukes)

1.75.) ARTHRITIS

You should be able to distinguish the clinical presentation of osteoarthritis and rheumatoid arthritis:

OSTEOARTHRITIS	RHEUMATOID ARTHRITIS (RA)
• women > men	• women 20~50 years
• loss of cartilage • narrowing of joint space • increased density of subchondral bone • osteophyte formation	• synovial membrane proliferation (pannus) • erosions of cartilage and subchondral bone
• knees, hips, spine • distal interphalangeal joints • joint stiffness after inactivity (e.g. sitting in chair) • Heberden's nodes	• starts in small joints • proximal interphalangeal joints • metacarpophalangeal joints • morning stiffness • soft tissue swelling • rheumatoid nodules (skin, valves..) • rheumatoid factor: anti IgG

 Heberden's nodes are osteophytes at the distal interphalangeal joints.

STILL'S DISEASE
• juvenile RA, acute febrile, no rheumatoid factors

PSORIATIC ARTHRITIS
• like RA, but absence of rheumatoid factors

FELTY'S SYNDROME
• polyarticular RA, splenomegaly, leukopenia, leg ulcers

1.76.) BONES

A) CONGENITAL:

	KEY FEATURES
osteogenesis imperfecta	• disorder of collagen synthesis • fractures • blue, thin sclera
osteopetrosis	• increased density • brittle bones • facial distortion due to bone overgrowth
achondroplasia	• autosomal dominant • defective cartilage synthesis • decreased epiphyseal formation • short limbs, normal size head and trunk

B) ACQUIRED: Diagnosis is made by X-ray and lab tests:

OSTEOPOROSIS	OSTEOMALACIA	PAGET'S
- thinned cortical bone - enlarged medullary cavity	- diffuse radiolucency	- bones enlarged and radiolucent
- normal Ca and phosphate - normal alk. phosphatase	- low Ca, low phosphate - high alk. phosphatase	- extremely high alkaline phosphatase
- decreased bone mass - estrogen deficiency - immobilization - Cushing's syndrome	- impaired mineralization - lack of Vit. D - chronic renal insufficiency	- excessive bone resorption with replacement

C) <u>PAGET'S DISEASE OF BONE</u>:

Gradual enlargement and deformation of bones (i.e *osteitis deformans*) with increased osteoclast and osteblast activity. Bones become brittle and have a characteristic X-ray appearance:

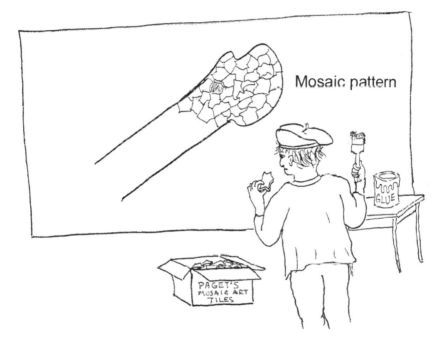

From Zaher: *Pathology Made Ridiculously Simple*, MedMaster, 2007

Don't confuse this with Paget's disease of the breast, which is an uncommon type of cancer around the nipple.

1.77.) CARTILAGE

Three types of cartilage differ by the composition of their extracellular matrix:

hyaline cartilage	**type II collagen** o joints o developing bones o joints o trachea/larynx o nose
elastic cartilage	**elastin** o ear
fibrocartilage	**type I collagen** o intervertebral disks o menisci

A) Benign Tumors:

	KEY FEATURES
osteochondroma	• developmental defect • exostosis at metaphyseal projections
enchondroma	• may develop into chondrosarcoma • cartilage within bone
chondroblastoma	• benign • femur, tibia, humerus epiphysis

B) Malignant Tumors:

	KEY FEATURES
chondrosarcoma	• malignant • spine, pelvic bones • slower growing than osteosarcoma

1.78.) BONE TUMORS

Diagnosis can often be made from location and typical X-ray appearance and should be considered together with the histopathology. You should know which tumors are benign and which are malignant:

A) Benign Tumors:

	KEY FEATURES
osteoma	• benign • skull
osteoid osteoma	• benign, painful • tibia or femur (diaphysis)
osteoblastoma	• like osteoid osteoma • larger but painless • may be malignant

B) Malignant Tumors:

	KEY FEATURES
osteosarcoma	• highly malignant • metaphysis of long bone (knee) • Codman's triangle
Ewing's sarcoma	• very aggressive • young males • pelvis, long bones • within marrow cavity • "onion skin" appearance

C) <u>Codman's Triangle</u>:

Triangular area of new subperiostal that is created when a tumor, most typically an osteosarcoma, raises the periosteum from the bone:

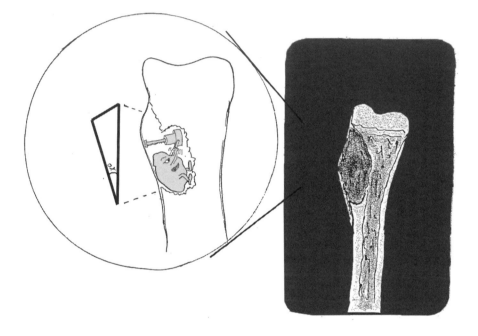

From Zaher: *Pathology Made Ridiculously Simple*, MedMaster, 2007

1.79.) MUSCULAR DYSTROPHIES

Dystrophies cause progressive weakness of select muscle groups.
Unfortunately, the most severe form is also the most common one:

	KEY FEATURES
Duchenne	**X linked** **absent dystrophin protein** • most severe • pelvic girdle weakness • pseudohypertrophy of calves
Becker	**X linked** **abnormal dystrophin protein** • less severe than Duchenne • may walk until age 20-25
limb girdle	**autosomal recessive** • late onset
facioscapulohumeral	**autosomal dominant** • late onset
myotonic	**autosomal dominant** • late onset • limb involvement is distal • inability to voluntarily relax muscle

Gower's sign: *When trying to stand up the child uses its hands to "climb up" his/her own body.*

<u>Clinical features (Duchenne)</u>:
• presents in boys age 3-7
• proximal muscle weakness → waddling gait
• pseudohypertrophy: fatty and fibrous infiltration of calve muscle
• increased serum CPK

1.80.) BRAIN TUMORS

Try to get a "feel" for which ones are relatively benign and which ones are severe:

		KEY FEATURES
Neural Tube	astrocytoma	• slow growing, M > F
	glioblastoma	• always fatal, M > F
	medulloblastoma	• children, M > F
	oligodendroblastoma	• rare, M = F slow growing, seizures
Neural Crest	meningioma	• from arachnoid, benign, F > M "whorling pattern" psammoma bodies
	Schwannoma	• acoustic neurinoma, F > M a/w von Recklinghausen's
	neurofibroma	• fibroblasts and Schwann cells, benign usually von Recklinghausen's
Ectoderm	craniopharyngioma	• most common supratentorial tumor in children, compresses optic nerve
	pituitary adenoma	• 60% prolactin (chromophobe) • 10% growth hormone (eosinophil) • 10% ACTH (basophil)
Mesoderm	lymphoma	• B cells, periventricular
	lipoma	• "egg shell" appearance
	hemangioblastoma	

1.81.) CNS DEGENERATION

Alzheimer's is the most common degenerative disease of the CNS. It's pathological features are (1.) diffuse cortical atrophy, (2.) senile plaques (β-amyloid protein), and (3.) neurofibrillary tangles (cytoplasmic deposit of tau protein). Compare with the less common degenerative diseases of the CNS:

	KEY FEATURES ◀
Pick's	• lobar atrophy • mainly frontal and temporal
Parkinson's	• bradykinesia, rigidity, resting tremor • dopamine depletion (caudate, putamen) • **Lewy bodies** (spherical inclusions in melanin-depleted neurons of the substantia nigra)
ALS	• rapidly progressive • degeneration of corticospinal tract (UMN) • degeneration of α-motoneurons (LMN)
Huntington's	• chorea, athetoid movements • atrophy of caudate, putamen and frontal cortex
Friedreich's ataxia	• autosomal recessive • pes cavus • loss of proprioception • tremors, Babinski reflex • spinal cord atrophy • (spinocerebellar, corticospinal, post. columns)

Upper motor neuron lesions: spasticity, increased tendon reflexes
Lower motor neuron lesions: paralysis, fasciculations, absent tendon reflexes

1.82.) DEMYELINATING DISEASES

Myelin sheaths are composed of lipoproteins and formed by the oligodendroglia (CNS) or Schwann cells (peripherally). Congenital metabolic disorders affect the developing myelination and results in severe neurological deficits.

Demyelination occurring in later life can be repaired by the glia. This explains for example the frequent exacerbations and remissions seen in multiple sclerosis.

	KEY FEATURES
multiple sclerosis	• onset at age 20-40 • a/w cool, temperate climate • oligoclonal bands
Devic's	• like MS, but **limited** to spinal chord and optical nerve
Guillain-Barré	• peripheral nerves (mainly motor) • autoimmune, often following viral infection
adrenoleukodystrophy	• X linked • accumulation of long chain cholesterols • blindness, ataxia • latent adrenal insufficiency
Schilder's	• focal demyelination in brain • children • visual, auditory, motor defects • variant of adrenoleukodystrophy

> ## Oligoclonal bands (CSF electrophoresis):
> o Multiple monoclonal gamma globulins.
> o Characteristic, but not entirely specific for MS.

1.83.) PITUITARY HYPERFUNCTION

ANTERIOR PITUITARY:

eosinophile cells	prolactin	**male:** decreased libido, impotence **female:** galactorrhea, amenorrhea, infertility
	GH	**prepubertal:** giantism **adults:** acromegaly
basophile cells	ACTH	**Cushing's disease** is the most common cause of Cushing's syndrome (except iatrogenic)

Classification according to staining properties is outdated since there is only an approximate relationship between hormones and cell staining.

While prolactin is mainly produced by eosinophil cells, prolactinomas are usually **chromophobe**!

1.84.) PITUITARY HYPOFUNCTION

Sheehan's syndrome (ischemic necrosis, often postpartum)	**panhypopituitarism:** • hypothyroidism • hypoadrenalism • hypogonadism
dwarfism	**a)** growth hormone deficiency **b)** lack of receptors (e.g. in pygmies)
eunuchoid hypogonadism, primary amenorrhea	gonadotropin deficiency (common!)

1.85.) ADRENAL ADENOMAS/CARCINOMAS

The adrenal gland has 2 distinct components: The cortex producing steroids and the medulla, derived from the neural crest, producing epinephrine and norepinephrine.

cortex: adenoma	most adenomas do <u>not</u> produce steroids **Conn**: mineralocorticoids ↑ **Cushing**: glucocorticoids ↑ **Virilization**: androgens ↑
cortex: carcinoma	much rarer than adenomas, but if they occur they usually produce hormones!
medulla: pheochromocytoma	**10%** extra-adrenal **10%** bilateral **10%** malignant
neuroblastoma	common tumor in children < 5 years from medulla or sympathetic chain ganglia

CONN: • hypernatremia → hypervolemia → high blood pressure
          • potassium loss → muscle weakness

CUSHING: • "moon face", "buffalo hump"
            • truncal obesity
            • skin striae
            • osteoporosis
            • low glucose tolerance

Mineral corticoids	zona **G**lomerulosa
Glucocorticoids	zona **F**asciculata
Androgens	zona **R**eticularis

"The deeper you go the sweeter it gets!"

1.86.) THYROID

Like the adrenals, the thyroid gland also has 2 distinct components: (1.) follicle cells produce T4 and T3, (2.) parafollicular C-cells make calcitonin. T3 is derived by removal of iodine from T4 in the blood and is much more potent!

		KEY FEATURES
hyperthyroidism:	Graves' (diffuse toxic goiter)	• lymphocytes • small follicles • little colloid
	Plummer's (nodular toxic goiter)	• hyperplasia, hypertrophy • colloid accumulation
hypothyroidism:	diffuse simple goiter (iodine deficiency)	• hyperplasia, hypertrophy
	Hashimoto's	• lymphocytes, plasma cells • atrophic follicles • little colloid
	Riedel's	• fibrous replacement
euthyroid:	De Quervain's	• viral • leakage of colloid • granulomas

"SICK EUTHYROID" SYNDROME
• Many patients with severe illness, trauma or stress have low T3 and low T4, but clinically no signs of hypothyroidism.
• TSH is also normal in these cases.

1.87.) THYROID TUMORS

		KEY FEATURES
benign:	follicular adenoma	• very common • most are cold nodules
malignant:	papillary CA	• younger patients • a/w radiation exposure • Psammoma bodies
	follicular CA	• adenomatous pattern
	anaplastic CA	• undifferentiated • poor prognosis
	medullary CA	• parafollicular (C cells)

 Medullary CA of the thyroid is often a/w MEN type II.

• **Papillary carcinoma** is more **common** than follicular carcinoma.
• **Follicular carcinoma** is more **aggressive** than papillary carcinoma.

1.88.) <u>PARATHYROIDS</u>

Derived from the 3rd and 4th pharyngeal pouches, these glands produce PTH. PTH acts on bone osteoclasts and mobilizes calcium.

	KEY FEATURES
hyperparathyroidism	<u>**primary**</u> adenoma *** <u>**secondary**</u> chronic renal failure Vit. D deficiency
hypoparathyroidism	• thyroidectomy *** • DiGeorge's syndrome ➢ **PTH low** ➢ **Ca^{2+} low**
pseudohypo...	• receptor defect • short stature • short metacarpal bones ➢ **PTH elevated** ➢ **Ca^{2+} low**
pseudopseudohypo...	• same physical appearance as in pseudohypoparathyroidism ➢ **PTH normal** ➢ **Ca^{2+} levels normal**

*** most common causes, respectively

RENAL OSTEODYSTROPHY
chronic renal failure→ decreased phosphate excretion
> → phosphate binds ionized calcium in serum
> → hypocalcemia
> → increased PTH
> → bone demineralization

TX: Aluminum may be used to bind phosphate.

1.89.) DIABETES MELLITUS

Most common endocrine disease → serious morbidity

A) PRIMARY DIABETES:

IDDM (Type I)	NIDDM (Type II)	MODY
• not so common	• very common	• rare
• juvenile onset • prone to ketoacidosis	• adult onset • not prone to ketoacidosis	• juvenile onset
• viral etiology?	• inadequate insulin secretion • obesity, insulin resistance	• glucokinase defect (glucose sensor)
• weak genetic predisposition [1] (HLA DR 3, DR4)	• strong genetic predisposition [2]	
• auto-immune (islet cell antibodies)	• hyalinization of islets	
• decreased number of β-cells		

[1] <50% concordance   [2] 100% concordance in monozygotic twins

B) SECONDARY DIABETES:

hemochromatosis	chronic pancreatitis, pancreas carcinoma
"bronze diabetes"	→ islet cell destruction

Gestational diabetes: *1-3% of women develop diabetes during pregnancy. This induces excessive fetal insulin secretion and increases the risk of birth trauma (increased fetal weight due to the metabolic effects of insulin). Usually glucose tolerance returns to normal after delivery, but 30% of women with gestational diabetes develop overt diabetes mellitus within 5 years.*

1.90.) MULTIPLE ENDOCRINE NEOPLASIA

MEN is inherited autosomal dominant with variable penetrance. MEN Type 1 is due to loss of a tumor suppressor gene. Neoplasia arises when the second, healthy allele of this gene mutates.

MEN Type 1	MEN Type 2A	MEN Type 2B
• adrenal <u>cortex</u> • pituitary • parathyroid • pancreas (gastrinoma)	• adrenal <u>medulla</u> • thyroid medulla • parathyroid	• adrenal <u>medulla</u> • thyroid medulla • mucosal neuromas • marfanoid features
"pity-para-pan"	"para-medullary-medulla"	

CLINICAL PRESENTATIONS

MEN 1:
- (90%) primary hyperparathyroidism → hypercalcemia
- (70%) gastrin → Zollinger-Ellison syndrome → peptic ulcers
- (60%) pituitary tumors → visual disturbances
  - (sometimes produce GH → acromegaly)

MEN 2A:
- (100%) medullary carcinoma of thyroid (bilateral)
  - → early diagnosis is essential!
- (50%) benign pheochromocytoma (bilateral)
  - → hypertensive crisis (headache, sweating, palpitations)
- (20%) primary hyperparathyroidism → hypercalcemia

Hypercalcemia is either asymptomatic or may produce kidney stones.

1.91.) SKIN TUMORS

Skin cancer is the most common cancer in the US and directly related to sun-exposure. 80% of these are basal cell carcinomas with very low metastatic potential.

A) BENIGN:

	KEY FEATURES
seborrheic keratosis	• brownish/gray, scaly, greasy
keratoacanthoma	• rapidly growing pink papula • looks like squamous cell carcinoma but is benign
actinic keratosis	• crusty red papule, premalignant

B) MALIGNANT:

	KEY FEATURES
basal cell carcinoma	• pearly, gray papule
squamous cell carcinoma	• erythematous, scaly or oozing ulcer • Bowen's disease: squamous CA in situ
melanoma	• brown, black, red, white, purple, irregular borders • **lentigo maligna:** grows horizontally • **nodular melanoma:** grows vertically

---

The "ABC" of melanoma
A - asymmetric lesion
B - borders irregular
C - color variations
D - diameter increasing

1.92.) OTHER SKIN DISEASES

Spend a day with a dermatology atlas and learn to recognize these:

	KEY FEATURES
pemphigus	• vesicles on mucosa • auto antibodies against intercellular junctions of keratinocytes
pemphigoid	• like pemphigus, but larger bullae on abdomen and groin
impetigo	• honey colored crust, superficial skin infection • *Staphylococcus* or β-hemolytic *Streptococci*
pityriasis	• (viral cause?) • herald patch → spreads along flexural lines
rosacea	• large, red nose

	KEY FEATURES
xanthoma	• hyperlipidemia, foamy histocytes
capillary hemangioma	• "salmon patches" and stork bites *spontaneously regresses* • "strawberry hemangiomas" *initially grows, later regresses*
cavernous hemangioma	• "port-wine stain", a/w Sturge-Weber *does not resolve spontaneously*
café-au-lait spots	• a/w von neurofibromatosis
vitiligo	• irregular depigmentation

95

1.93.) TOXINS

	PATHOLOGY
cadmium	"honeycomb" pneumonitis
cobalt	cardiomyopathy
chromium	lung cancer
lead	inhibits heme synthesis renal tubular acidosis
mercury	neurotoxic ("Minamata disease") proximal tubular necrosis
arsenic	lung cancer
asbestos	mesothelioma
aromatic amines	bladder cancer
benzene	leukemia
vinyl chloride	liver angiosarcoma
α-amanitin	fulminant hepatitis
CO	forms carboxyhemoglobin [1]
cyanide	inhibits mitochondrial cytochromes $\rightarrow$ loss of O_2 utilization

[1] *do not confuse with methemoglobin, which contains oxidized Fe^{3+}*

High-Yield Pictures

Be able to recognize the following pictures:

MICROSCOPIC:

- **Amyloid:** birefringence
- **Red blood cells:** microcytic hypochrome versus macrocytic megaloblastic
  - target cells
  - sickle cells
- **White blood cells:** ALL versus AML
- **Reed-Sternberg cell** (Hodgkin's disease)
- **Barrett's esophagus:** metaplasia
- **Granulomas:** caseating (TBC) versus non-caseating (foreign body)
- **Lung:** acid fast bacilli
  - Aspergillus,
  - Pneumocystis carinii (silver stain)
- **Lung:** oat cell carcinoma
- **Breast:** normal versus fibroadenoma versus cancer
- **Kaposi sarcoma**
- **Teratoma:** skin, teeth, neural tissue etc.
- **Giant cell arteritis**
- **Bacterial pneumonia**
- **Kidneys:** hypertensive change
- **Kidney immunofluorescence:** linear pattern (Goodpasture's syndrome)
  - granular pattern (membranous GN)
  - mesangial pattern (IgA nephropathy)
- **Colon:** adenomatous polyp versus adenocarcinoma
- **Liver:** hepatitis, fatty degeneration
- **Ovary:** Krukenberg tumor (signet ring cells)
- **Cervix:** carcinoma in situ
- **Pap smear:** dysplastic cell versus glycogen rich normal cells
- **CNS:** Alzheimer's disease: neurofibrillary tangles, plaques
  - Parkinson's disease: depigmentation of substantia nigra

MACROSCOPIC:

- **Cardiac hypertrophy:** eccentric versus concentric hypertrophy
- **Breast carcinoma:** (mammography)
- **Lung:** Ghon complex (X-ray)
- **Gall-bladder:** stone types
- **Hydatidiform mole**
- **Pituitary adenoma** (X-ray of sella turcica)
- **Brain:** atrophy of cortex
     atrophy of caudate nucleus

MICROBIOLOGY

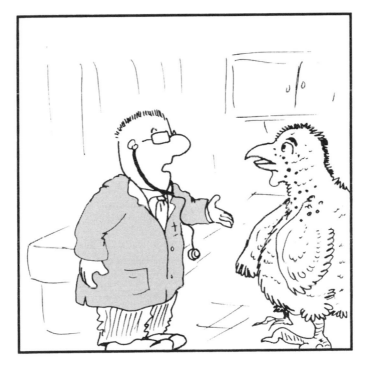

"It could be chickenpox, but then all these
viruses look similar."

Part A : General Microbiology

2.1.) GRAM STAIN

Stains take advantage of special properties in the cell walls from different organisms. The most famous is Gram, separating bacteria into 3 classes:
1. **Gram+ bacteria** are rich in peptidoglycan and retain violet dye.
2. **Gram- bacteria** are poor in peptidoglycan but counterstain with red dye.
3. Bacteria that do not stain with either dye, requiring "special stains".

> 1. Crystal violet dye (plus iodine) <u>stains</u> all bacterial cell walls.
> 2. Alcohol <u>extracts</u> blue dye from lipid-rich, thin-walled gram-negative bacteria.
> 3. Red dye <u>counterstains</u> decolorized gram-negative bacteria.

2.2.) SPECIAL STAINS

	USED FOR:
Ziehl Neelsen	stains acid fast bacteria red
India ink	cryptococcus
Giemsa	blood smears
PAS	glycogen, mucopolysaccharides
Prussian blue	iron
Congo red	amyloid
osmic acid	for electron microscopy

2.3.) <u>NORMAL FLORA</u>

Normal flora is all microorganisms that are found in particular sites in healthy people. Often, they have a symbiotic relationship with the host:
- They stimulate the immune system of newborns.
- They interfere with colonization by pathogenic strains.

	NORMAL FLORA	POTENTIAL PATHOGENS
skin	*Staph. epidermidis*	*Staph. aureus*
nasopharynx	*Strep. viridans* anaerobes	*Strep. pneumoniae* N. meningitides H. influenzae
mouth	*Strep. viridans*	*Candida albicans*
colon	*E. coli*	*Bacteroides fragilis* enterococci
vagina	*Lactobacillus* Streptococci	*Candida albicans*

<u>*Clinical examples*</u>*:*
- *Risk of endocarditis after dental procedures (Strep. viridans).*
- *Pseudomembranous colitis following administration of broad-spectrum antibiotics (Cl. difficile usually suppressed by endogenous flora).*

2.4.) <u>CELL WALLS</u>

all bacteria (except mycoplasma)	**inner layer of cell wall: peptidoglycans** • thick in gram-positives • thin in gram-negatives
gram-positive	**outer layer of cell wall**: teichoic acid
gram-negative	**outer layer of cell wall**: lipopolysaccharides (=endotoxins)[1] • outer cell membrane (lipid bilayer) • porins
mycobacteria	• mycolic acid in cell wall (resists decoloration of gram-stain)
mycoplasma	• has no cell wall • only bacterium whose membrane contains cholesterol!
spores	• dipicolinic acid (keratin coat) → resistance to heat, dehydration and chemicals

[1] *the space between outer membrane and cell membrane contains*
β-lactamase (degrades penicillins).

<u>CELL CAPSULE</u>
• composed of polysaccharides
• determines virulence
• capsular antigens determine species
• vaccines are made against capsular antigens

Penicillin Attacks Peptidoglycans:

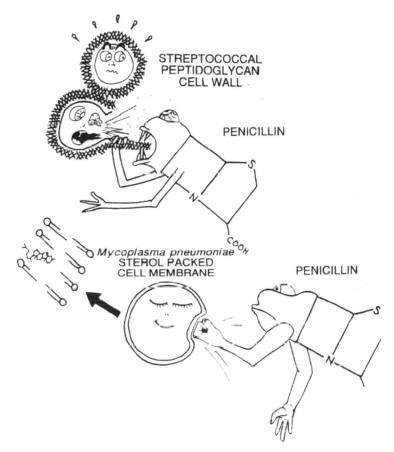

2.5.) TOXINS

Exotoxins are made by Gram+ and Gram- bacteria, are proteins and can be neutralized by antibodies (=antitoxins). Endotoxins are lipopolysaccharides from Gram- bacteria and are poorly antigenic.

ENDOTOXINS	• lipopolysaccharides • non-specific • TNF, IL-1 → fever, shock • poor antigen • heat **stable**
EXOTOXINS	• polypeptides • specific • toxoids used as vaccine • usually **heat labile**
tetanus toxin	• blocks release of glycine → muscle spasms
botulinum toxin	• blocks release of ACh → muscle paralysis
diphtheria toxin	• inhibits protein synthesis (ADP-ribosylation of EF-2)
alpha toxin	*Staph. aureus* • hemolysis, necrosis, cell death
toxic shock syndrome toxin	*Staph. aureus* • induces cytokines → anaphylactic shock
cholera toxin	• stimulates adenylate cyclase (activates G_s)
pertussis toxin	• stimulates adenylate cyclase (inhibits G_i)
enterotoxin	*E. coli* • **heat labile:** stimulates adenylate cyclase • **heat stable:** stimulates guanylate cyclase

2.6.) <u>O_2-REQUIREMENTS</u>

- Aerobes require O_2 and cannot ferment.
- Obligate anaerobes ferment and are killed by O_2.
- Microaerophilics grow best at low O_2 but also can grow without O_2.

obligate aerobe	• *M. tuberculosis* • *Pseudomonas aeruginosa* • *Nocardia*
microaerophilic	• *Campylobacter jejuni* • *Brucella abortus*
obligate anaerobe	• *Clostridium* • *Actinomyces*
facultative anaerobe	most others

Reactivation of tuberculosis usually appears in the upper lobes of the lung, where the ventilation/perfusion (V/Q) ratio is highest!

2.7.) MOST COMMON CAUSES

Many times, treatment cannot await the microbial lab results.
Choose your therapy based on your best guess of most common causes:

common cold	rhino viruses
pharyngitis, laryngitis	viral > bacterial (ß-hemolyzing Streptococci)
tonsillitis	ß-hemolyzing Streptococci
sinusitis	*Strep. pneumoniae, Staph. aureus*
otitis media	*Strep. pneumoniae, Hemophilus influenza*
bronchitis	*Hemophilus influenza, Strep. pneumoniae*
pneumonia - infants	**RSV**
- young adults	***Mycoplasma***
- elderly	***Strep. pneumoniae***
bacterial meningitis	
- neonates	***E. coli, Strep. agalactia, Listeria***
- adults	***Neisseria meningitidis > Strep. pneum.***
- elderly	**Strep. pneumoniae > Neisseria mening.**
aseptic meningitis	enteroviruses, arboviruses (Summer!)
endocarditis	*Strep. viridans*
carbuncle	*Staph. aureus*
sepsis (catheterized patient)	*Staph. aureus, Candida*
sepsis (burn wounds)	*Pseudomonas aeruginosa*
diarrhea - children	**Rotavirus**
- adults (US)	***Campylobacter***
- travelers	***E. coli, shigella, salmonella***
genital ulcer	herpes > syphilis
urethritis	*chlamydia > gonococcus*
cystitis	*E. coli*

Part B : Bacteria

2.8.) STAPHYLOCOCCI
(catalase +)

Staphylococci are Gram+ cocci that grow in grape-like clusters. Catalase is an enzyme that converts $2\ H_2O_2 \rightarrow 2\ H_2O + O_2$. Its presence distinguishes Staphylococci from Streptococci. Coagulase is specific for *Staph. aureus* and causes blood clotting.

	COAGULASE	NOVOBIOCIN	DISEASES
S. aureus	+		skin infections osteomyelitis endocarditis toxic shock syndrome food poisoning
S. epidermidis	-	sensitive	infections following: instrumentation implants etc.
S. saprophyticus	-	insensitive	urinary tract infections

FAMOUS EXOTOXINS
- Enterotoxin A-F → diarrhea
- Toxic shock syndrome toxin → anaphylaxis
- Exfoliatin → scalded skin (hands and feet)
- Alpha toxin → tissue necrosis

Staph. aureus:
- *Colonizes anterior nares of most people.*
- *Community cases usually due to poor hygiene.*
- *Hospital cases usually involve patients who underwent invasive procedures.*
- *Easily spread by hands of medical personnel.*

2.9.) STREPTOCOCCI

(catalase -)

Streptococci are Gram+ cocci that grow in chains. Compared to staphylococci, they grow better on enriched media and require a narrower temperature range. When grown on blood agar, they cause a characteristic pattern of RBC hemolysis which allows for a rough classification. Lancefield antigens determine the group and correlate better with pathogenicity.

	KEY FEATURES
ß-hemolytic streptococci complete hemolysis (clear halo)	***Strept. pyogenes* (Group A)** [1] → pharyngitis → acute rheumatic fever → bacitracin sensitive **other Strept. (Groups B-T)** [1] → neonatal sepsis → meningitis → bacitracin insensitive

[1] *C-antigen, cell-wall (=Lancefield antigen)*

"Strep throat":
- *acute sore throat*
- *malaise, fever (39° - 40°)*
- *yellow exudates on tonsils*
- *may need bacterial culture to distinguish from viral pharyngitis*

	KEY FEATURES
α-hemolytic streptococci incomplete hemolysis (green halo)	***Pneumococcus*** → "classic" lobar pneumonia • capsule determines virulence (over 80 distinct serotypes) • bile soluble (lysis) • Optochin sensitive ***Strept. viridans*** → endocarditis • bile insoluble • Optochin insensitive
γ-hemolytic streptococci no hemolysis	**Enterococci (Group D)** → urinary tract infections

Enterococci are more resistant to antibiotics than other streptococci.

FAMOUS EXOTOXINS
- Streptokinase
- Streptodornase (DNAse)
- Hyaluronidase
- Erythrogenic toxin
- Streptolysin O
- Streptolysin S

2.10.) NEISSERIA

bean-shaped, gram-negative diplococci

There are only 2 Neisseria species that cause human disease:

	KEY FEATURES
Meningococcus	• **has capsule** • ferments maltose • meningitis (infants 6-24 months) [1] • Waterhouse-Friderichsen syndrome • Gram stain of CSF is diagnostic ➤ *TX:* penicillin *G*

Gonococcus	• **has pilus**
	• does not ferment maltose
	
	• **male** : dysuria
	               purulent discharge
	• **female:** endocervical infections
	               salpingitis
	               infertility
	
	➤ *TX:* - almost all resistant to penicillin
	       - ceftriaxone is drug of choice [2]

[1] *"natural immunity" protects during the first 6 months of life, due to maternal IgG crossing the placenta.*

[2] *add tetracycline for coexisting C. trachomatis infection!*

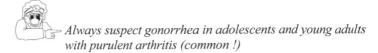 *Always suspect gonorrhea in adolescents and young adults with purulent arthritis (common !)*

Neisseria as seen under the microscope:

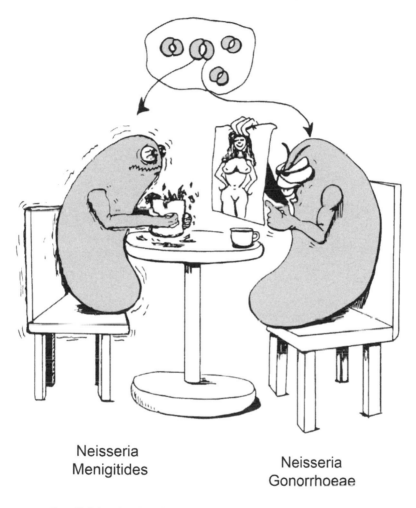

Neisseria
Menigitides

Neisseria
Gonorrhoeae

From Gladwin and Trattler: *Clinical Microbiology Made Ridiculously Simple*, MedMaster, 2008

2.11.) BACILLI

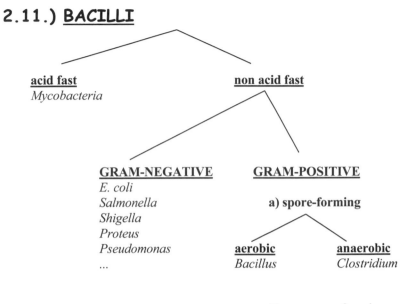

acid fast
Mycobacteria

non acid fast

GRAM-NEGATIVE
E. coli
Salmonella
Shigella
Proteus
Pseudomonas
...

GRAM-POSITIVE

a) spore-forming

aerobic
Bacillus

anaerobic
Clostridium

b) non spore-forming

Listeria
Corynebacteria

*"Bacilli" refers to any rod-shaped bacteria. The genus **Bacillus** specifically refers to **Gram+ spore-forming aerobic rods**.*

2.12.) <u>GRAM-POSITIVE BACILLI</u>

	AEROBE	TOXINS	SPORES	
Bacillus anthracis	+	+	+	→ anthrax → woolsorter's disease → "fried rice" poisoning
Coryne-bacterium	+	+	-	→ diphtheria pseudomembranes Loeffler's telluride "Chinese characters"
Listeria	+	-	-	→ sepsis, meningitis neonates & immunosuppressed "Chinese characters" + motile!
Clostridium	-	+	+	→ tetanus → botulism → gas gangrene (α-toxin) → food poisoning (reheated meat) → pseudomembranous colitis
Lactobacillus	-	-	-	protects GI and vagina prefers acidic pH < 4.5

<u>PSEUDOMEMBRANOUS COLITIS</u>
(the usual suspects):
➤ clindamycin
➤ ampicillin
➤ cephalosporins

2.13.) <u>CLOSTRIDIA</u>

Clostridia are anaerobe spore-forming rods found in the soil, especially when fertilized with animal excrements.

	KEY FEATURES
Cl. botulinum	• motile • types A-G (antigenically different exotoxins)
Cl. tetani	• motile • 10 types (flagellar antigen) • but all have the same exotoxin

Cl. perfringens	• non-motile
	
	• α-toxin = lecithinase
	  → gas gangrene (soldiers)
	
	• enterotoxin (heat labile)
	  → food poisoning (reheated meat stews)

<u>Signs of Tetanus:</u>

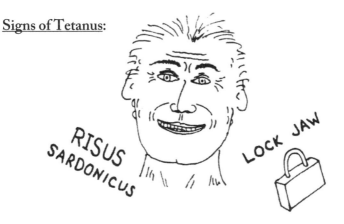

RISUS SARDONICUS

LOCK JAW

From Gladwin and Trattler: *Clinical Microbiology Made Ridiculously Simple*, MedMaster, 2008

BOTULISM

- *Cl. Botulinum* spores are highly resistant to heat, but toxins are not.
- Proper canning and heating of food prevents botulism.
- Nausea, vomiting and abdominal cramps usually precede the neurological symptoms: Dry mouth, diplopia, loss of pupillary reflexes, followed by descending paralysis and respiratory failure.

TETANUS

- Toxin enters the CNS along the peripheral nerves
- Incubation period 5~10 days
- Stiffness of the jaws, difficulty swallowing, fever, headache
- *Risus sardonicus*: fixed "smile" and elevated eyebrows
- Severe spasms of neck, back and abdominal muscles
- Intact sensorium and CSF

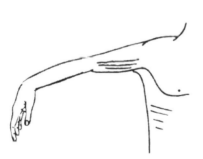 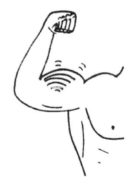

BOTULISM **TETANUS**

From Gladwin and Trattler: *Clinical Microbiology Made Ridiculously Simple*, MedMaster, 2008

2.14.) ENTEROBACTERIACEAE
(facultative anaerobe gram-negative rods)

Enterobacteriaceae are the most common cause of UTI and a major cause of diarrhea. They inhabit the lower GI tract of humans and animals and survive easily in free nature.

> **5 major genera.** All look the same, some are motile, some are not. Differentiated by cultural appearance and biochemical activities. Subtyping is done by serology.

	LAB FEATURES	CLINICAL FEATURES
E. coli	**motile** **lactose +**	→ most common cause of UTI → neonatal meningitis [1]
Salmonella (1,500 species)	motile lactose - only *S. typhi* produces gas	**food poisoning** • poultry products • incubation 1~2 days **enteric fever** (typhoid, paratyphoid) • incubation 10~14 days
Shigella	non-motile lactose - no gas	**dysenteriae** (serious) **flexneri, boydii, sonnei** (mild) • watery diarrhea followed by fever, bloody stools and cramping

[1] *maternal IgM are too big and do NOT cross placenta → no protection*

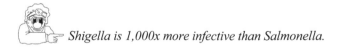 *Shigella is 1,000x more infective than Salmonella.*

> ### TREATMENT OF SALMONELLA INFECTIONS
> **gastroenteritis:** fluid replacement, no antibiotics
> **typhoid:**   chloramphenicol, ampicillin

Shigella attacks and invades gastrointestinal epithelium:

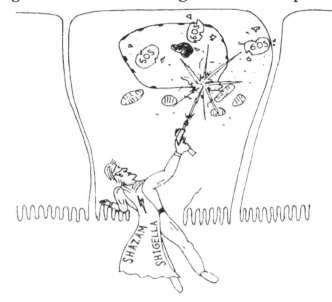

Enterobacteriacae exchange plasmids via conjugation:

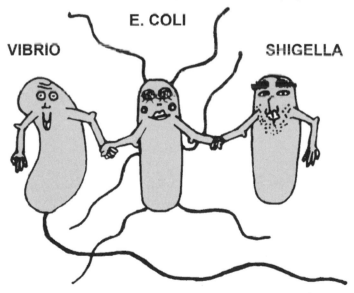

From Gladwin and Trattler: *Clinical Microbiology Made Ridiculously Simple*, MedMaster, 2008

2.15.) <u>MORE ENTEROBACTERIACEAE</u>

	LAB FEATURES	CLINICAL FEATURES
Proteus [1]	motile urease	**urinary tract infections** urease-production → ammonium calculi *Proteus* does NOT cause gastroenteritis
Klebsiella	non-motile encapsulated	**Community acquired:** - indistinguishable from "classic" lobar pneumonia - "currant jelly" sputum **Hospital acquired:** - UTI - respiratory tract infections - wound infections - **resistant to many antibiotics !!!**

[1] *has antigens that cross-react with anti-rickettsial antibodies*
(Weil-Felix reaction)

> **K-antigen:** capsule
> **H-antigen:** flagella
> **O-antigen:** surface

Patients recovering from Salmonella gastroenteritis can shed the
organism for many weeks or months. Beware of chronic carriers
who handle foods!

	KEY FEATURES
Bacteroides fragilis anaerobic	• most common cause of gram-negative abdominal infections • forms abscesses in organs or deep tissues ➤ *TX: metronidazole*
Vibrio cholera comma-shaped	• rice-watery diarrhea (non bloody) ➤ *TX: tetracycline*
Vibrio parahaemolyticus comma-shaped	• diarrhea from raw seafood (Sushi) ➤ *self-limited*
Campylobacter jejuni curved rods	• watery, foul smelling stools later may become bloody • most common cause of diarrhea in US ➤ *TX: erythromycin, aminoglycoside*
Helicobacter pylori very similar to Campylobacter (but urease +)	• gastritis • peptic ulcer • MALT lymphoma ➤ *TX: metronidazole + tetracycline + bismuth* *(three drug regimen)*

 CHOLERA TOXIN:

ADP-ribosylates stimulatory G_S protein (locks it in the "on"-state)
→ permanent activation of adenylate cyclase
→ secretory diarrhea

2.16.) <u>GRAM- BACILLI (ZOONOTIC)</u>

	KEY FEATURES
Yersinia pestis bipolar staining	**bubonic plague** rodents → fleas → humans large, very tender lymph nodes **pulmonary plague** humans → humans ➤ *TX: streptomycin, tetracycline*
Pasteurella	• wound infections (dog and cat bites) • cellulitis, osteomyelitis ➤ *TX: penicillin G*
Brucella	undulating fever • Br. abortus (cattle) • Br. melitensis (goats and sheep) • Br. suis (hogs) ➤ *TX: tetracycline, gentamycin*
Francisella	tularemia • rabbits → ticks → humans • influenza-like • large, tender lymph nodes ➤ *TX: streptomycin*

Plague: Infection in a human occurs when a person is bitten by a flea that has been infected by biting a rodent that itself has been infected by the bite of a flea carrying *Yersinia pestis*. This way the disease is transmitted from wild rodents to domestic rodents to humans under conditions of crowding and poverty.

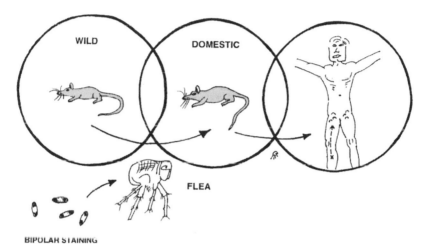

From Gladwin and Trattler: *Clinical Microbiology Made Ridiculously Simple*, MedMaster, 2008

Plague ("Black Death") *killed 25 million people in Europe in the 14th Century. Today, 30-40 cases are reported annually in the US. Bubonic plague has up to 75% mortality, pneumonic plague has 100% mortality if untreated. Avoid sick or dead wild rodents!*

2.17.) OTHER GRAM- BACILLI

	KEY FEATURES
Pseudomonas	• easily survives in un-sterile water • musty odor, greenish bluish pus • common wound infection (especially burns) • pneumonia, UTI ➤ *resists most antibiotics and disinfectants !!!*
Hemophilus	• very small bacterium • requires blood (chocolate agar) for culture • dramatic decrease since vaccination • *H. influenza* : bronchitis, meningitis • *H. ducreyi* : chancroid
Bordetella	• pertussis toxin → whooping cough ➤ *TX: erythromycin (best during catarrhal stage!)*
Legionella *(aerobe)*	• gram-negative cell wall, but stains only faintly • found in any stagnant water • atypical pneumonia [1] • no cold agglutinins (unlike mycoplasma) ➤ *TX: erythromycin*

[1] *clinical spectrum ranges from mild, self-limited to fatal Legionnaire's disease.*

PERTUSSIS TOXIN:
   ADP-ribosylates inhibitory Gi protein(locks it in the "off"-state)
   → permanent activation of adenylate cyclase

2.18.) MYCOBACTERIA

About half of the World population is infected with *M. tuberculosis*. 30 million people have active disease. Related to poverty, overcrowding and poor hygiene.

	KEY FEATURES
M. tuberculosis	• slow respiratory infection • primary lesion: Ghon complex • most morbidity is due to reactivation
M. bovis	• unpasteurized milk • GI tuberculosis

M. leprae	• grows at lower temp. than *M. tuberculosis*
	• found in nasal secretions and skin lesions
	• **tuberculoid leprosy:** granulomas
	                     skin test positive
	• **lepromatous leprosy:** nodular skin lesions
	                     skin test negative [1]

Atypical ***M. avium-intracellulare***	 • clinically indistinguishable from tuberculosis • immunosuppressed patients (AIDS) ➤ *highly resistant to therapy !!!*
M. marinum	• causes tuberculosis in fish • "swimming pool granuloma" in humans

[1] *due to deficiency in cell-mediated immunity!*

TUBERCULOSIS

Ghon complex: primary lesion in lung + calcified hilar lymph node
reactivation: favors upper lobes of lung
liquefying necrosis → cavity formation
miliary TBC: due to hematogenous spread of tubercle bacilli
(lesions resemble millet seeds)

2.19.) HIGHER BACTERIA

- gram-positive rods
- filamentous, branching growth: were confused with fungi in the past
- cause indolent, slowly progressive diseases

	KEY FEATURES
Actinomyces anaerobe	• growths in normal mouth flora **Lump jaw** • following tooth extraction • inflammatory sinuses → discharge to surface • sulfur granules ➤ *TX: penicillin* *surgical drainage*
Nocardia aerobe	• growths in soil **Subcutaneous tissue infections** • following minor trauma (outdoors) **Pulmonary infections** • inhalation of dust or soil ➤ *TX: sulfonamides* *surgical drainage*

From Gladwin and Trattler: *Clinical Microbiology Made Ridiculously Simple*, MedMaster, 2008

2.20.) SPIROCHETES

	KEY FEATURES
T. pallidum	• syphilis • related diseases: Yaws, Bejel, Pinta ➢ *TX: penicillin G*
B. burgdorferi	• Lyme disease • tick bite (mainly east coast) *TX: doxycycline, ceftriaxone, amoxicillin*
B. recurrentis	• relapsing fever • antigens undergo variations → relapses • human → louse or tick → human ➢ *TX: tetracycline*
L. interrogans	• leptospirosis • sewers, water contaminated with <u>rat urine</u> • fever, jaundice, hemorrhage, uremia ➢ *TX: penicillin G*

LYME DISEASE

1.) primary lesion (3~30 days):   – at site of tick bite
                                            – expanding macule or papule with
                                                  central clearing *(erythema migrans)*

2.) second stage (weeks ~ months):   – cardiac AV block
                                            – fluctuating meningitis
                                            – facial palsy
                                            – peripheral neuropathy

3.) third stage (weeks ~ years):   – arthritis of large joints (knee)

2.21.) CHLAMYDIA

Intracellular bacterium that cannot make ATP and cannot live outside.
Cell wall does not contain peptidoglycans!

	KEY FEATURES
C. pneumoniae	• "walking pneumonia" in young adults ➤ *TX: tetracycline*

C. trachomatis	**different strains cause different diseases :**
	
	• **urethritis**
	  most common non-gonorrheal urethritis
	• **lymphogranuloma venereum**
	  large and tender inguinal lymph nodes
	  may drain pus through skin
	• **trachoma**
	  chronic conjunctivitis that leads to blindness
	
	➤ *TX: tetracycline*

C. psittaci	• **pneumonia** (sometimes plus hepatitis) from bird feces ➤ *TX: tetracycline*

 Giemsa stain shows typical cytoplasmic inclusions in epithelial cells.

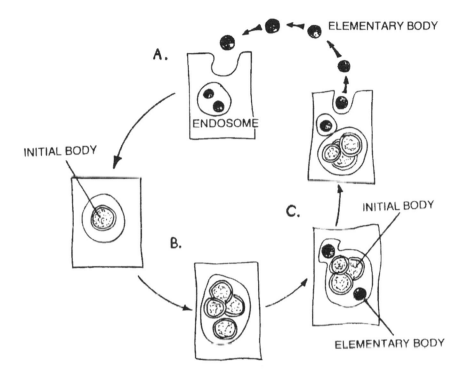

ELEMENTARY BODY

A.

ENDOSOME

INITIAL BODY

B.

C.

INITIAL BODY

ELEMENTARY BODY

From Gladwin and Trattler: *Clinical Microbiology Made Ridiculously Simple*, MedMaster, 2008

LIFE CYCLE OF CHLAMYDIAE

A Elementary body infects cell (attaches to cell membrane and enters the cell by endocytosis).

B Elementary body then transforms into a large initial body (= reticulate body = visible cytoplasmic inclusions).

C Initial body condenses and forms many new elementary bodies that are released when cell ruptures.

2.22.) RICKETTSIA

		VECTOR	RESERVOIR
Typhus: epidemic [1] **endemic** [2] **scrub** [3]	*R. prowazekii* *R. typhi* *R. tsutsugamushi*	lice fleas mite	humans rodents rodents
Rocky Mountain spotted fever	*R. rickettsiae*	ticks	dogs, rodents
Q fever	*C. burnetii*	transmitted by inhalation (slaughterhouses)	cattle, sheep
Trench fever	*R. quintana*	lice	humans

[1] *war, famine, crowding, infrequent bathing (no cases in US since WW II)*
[2] *murine typhus, 30–60 cases/year in US (mostly Texas)*
[3] *Southeast Asia, Japan*

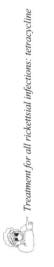

Treatment for all rickettsial infections: tetracycline

Rocky Mountain Spotted Fever:

- Fever
- Headache
- Conjunctival redness
- Rash that first appears on the wrists and later spreads to trunk

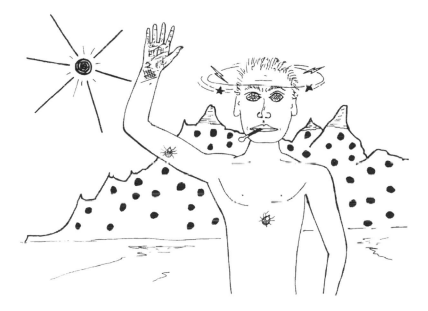

From Gladwin and Trattler: *Clinical Microbiology Made Ridiculously Simple*, MedMaster, 2008

Part C : Viruses

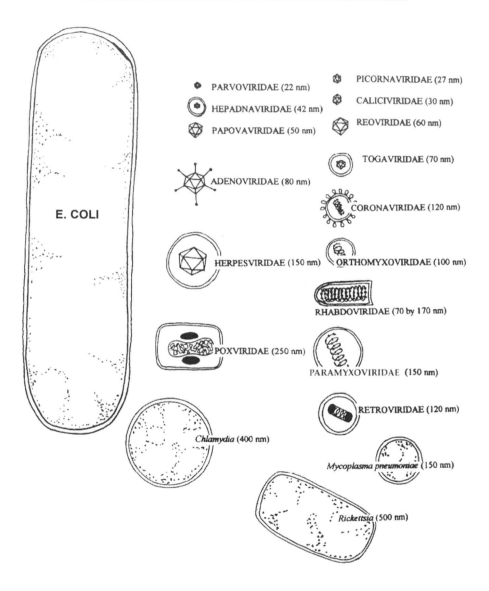

From Gladwin and Trattler: *Clinical Microbiology Made Ridiculously Simple*, MedMaster, 2008

2.23.) DNA VIRUSES

- ➤ All DNA viruses have a double stranded genome, except parvoviruses.
- ➤ All DNA viruses have an icosahedral nucleocapsid, except poxviruses.
- ➤ Pox are the largest and most complex viruses.

FAMILY	VIRUS	DISEASES
Parvo	B19	• erythema infectiosum, (5th disease) "slapped cheek" appearance
Papova	Papilloma	• genital warts → cervix carcinoma multiply in squamous cells
	JC	• leukoencephalopathy (in immunocompromised patients)
Adeno	~100 serotypes	• respiratory infections • atypical pneumonia ○ conjunctivitis ○ gastroenteritis ○ hemorrhagic cystitis
Pox	Variola	• smallpox , has been eradicated
	Vaccinia	• cowpox
	Molluscum contagiosum	• small pink warts of skin
Hepadna	HBV	• serum hepatitis B liver cell carcinoma

Vaccinia is serologically related to Variola, but the origin of this virus (recombinant of smallpox and cowpox?) is unknown.

2.24.) HERPES VIRUSES
(double stranded DNA)

All Herpes viruses produce an initial overt infection followed by a period of latency. Reactivation of virus in immunocompromised host results in recurrent infection.

VIRUS	DISEASES	during latency the virus rests in:
HSV1 HSV2	• mainly oral herpes • mainly genital herpes - both multiply in fibroblasts	trigeminal ganglion sacral DRG
VZV	• chickenpox, shingles	thoracolumbar DRG [1]
EBV	• infectious mononucleosis ○ Burkitt's lymphoma (Africa) ○ nasopharyngeal carcinoma (China)	B lymphocytes
CMV	• cytomegalic inclusion disease heterophil negative mononucleosis (no pharyngitis !)	leukocytes
HHV-6	• roseola (6th disease)	T lymphocytes
HHV-8	• Kaposi sarcoma	unknown

[1] *DRG = dorsal root ganglion: eruptions follow sensory nerve distribution!*

Chickenpox: lesions appear in <u>different</u> stages of evolution
(vesicular → pustular → crusts)

Smallpox: lesions appear in <u>same</u> stage of evolution

2.25.) <u>RNA VIRUSES</u>

80% of respiratory tract infections are viral. The most important are influenza (RNA), parainfluenza (RNA), rhinovirus (RNA) and adenovirus (DNA).

FAMILY	VIRUS	DISEASES
Picorna	**Rhino** Echo	• **common cold** • meningitis, URI, diarrhea
	Hepatitis A Polio	• infectious hepatitis A • paralysis (α-motoneuron)
	Coxsackie A	• herpangina • hand/foot/mouth disease
	Coxsackie B	• myocarditis • Bornholm disease
Reo	Rota	• gastroenteritis (children)
Orthomyxo	**Influenza A, B, C**	• **influenza** H antigen: hemagglutinin N antigen: neuraminidase
Paramyxo	Rubeola	• measles • encephalitis • SSPE
	Parainfluenza Mumps RSV	• **croup** (subglottitis) • parotitis, orchitis • bronchiolitis, pneumonia
Toga	Rubella Arbo	• German measles • encephalitis

ANTIGENIC DRIFT:	*"drift along"* (mutations within H_1N_1) - subtle changes of H or N antigens - caused by point mutations of viral RNA
ANTIGENIC SHIFT:	*"shift gears"* ($H_1N_2 \rightarrow H_1N_1$) - severe epidemics / pandemics - caused by gene recombination

2.26.) ARBO VIRUSES
(ARthropod BOrne)

Arboviruses cause seasonal disease transmitted by insects (arthropods). Reservoir are birds and small mammals.

FAMILY	VIRUS	DISEASES	VECTOR
Toga	**Alphavirus**	• EEE • WEE	mosquito
Flavi	**Flavivirus**	• St. Louis encephalitis • yellow fever • Dengue fever	mosquito
Bunya	**Bunyavirus**	• California encephalitis	mosquito
	Hantavirus	• fulminant respiratory infection	deer mice
Reo	**Orbivirus**	• Colorado tick fever	tick

Hantavirus *is an exception among Arboviruses: no arthropod vector!*

2.27.) SLOW VIRAL DISEASES OF CNS

Slowly progressing neurologic diseases due to viral persistence.

> ➤ personality changes
> ➤ intellectual deterioration
> ➤ autonomic or motor dysfunctions

AIDS dementia complex	HIV
subacute sclerosing panencephalitis	measles virus
progressive multifocal leukoencephalopathy	JC virus

2.28.) PRIONS

Prions are infectious proteins:
- o can be transmitted to other species (chimpanzees, mice etc.)
  by inoculation of infected brain tissue
- o are NOT transmitted by body secretions
  (no risk for medical personnel and care givers)
- o are NOT inactivated by formalin!

Kuru ("trembling disease")	humans
Creutzfeldt-Jakob	humans
Scrapie	sheep
BSE ("mad cow disease")	cattle

 Scrapie is not transmitted to humans. BSE may occasionally cause a variant of Creutzfeldt-Jacob disease.

2.29.) <u>RETROVIRUSES</u>

Single stranded RNA viruses encode a reverse transcriptase (RNA-dependent DNA polymerase that copies the virus genome into the host genome):

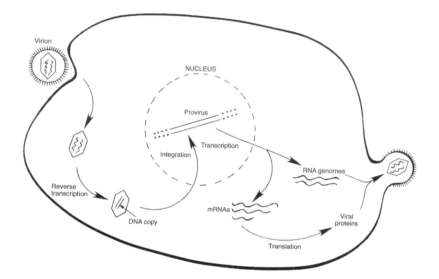

From *Sherris Medical Microbiology*, 3rd edition, p. 544, edited by Kenneth J. Ryan.
Copyright 1994 by Appleton&Lange, Norwalk, Connecticut. Used with permission.

Two main groups: (onco=tumor, lenti=slow)

oncoviruses	HTLV-1	adult T-cell leukemia
lentiviruses	HIV-1 HIV-2	AIDS

HTLV-1 simply activates existing cellular genes (c-onc = protooncogenes) resulting in malignant transformation.
Other retroviruses cause tumors (in animals) by expressing viral oncogenes (v-onc) or inserting promoters or enhancers in the vicinity of proto-oncogenes (c-onc).

2.30.) HIV

HIV is the causative agent of AIDS. HIV-1 is the most common and many subtypes have been found depending on geographic location. HIV-2 (West-Africa) is much less common and less virulent. It may give "false negative" on the usual ELISA test. The genome of HIV contains only 3 major genes: env, gag, and pol:

genome	• two identical single strands of RNA (both have positive polarity, cannot form double strand!)
env	• **gp41** : mediates cell fusion • **gp120** : binds to CD4 receptor (mutates rapidly !) gp = glycoproteins in lipid envelope
gag	• core capsid protein: **p24 (serologic marker)**
pol	• reverse transcriptase • integrase • protease
tat	• regulatory portion of genome • increases rate of transcription • also suppresses synthesis of class I MHC proteins

<u>Tests for HIV antibodies:</u>

ELISA: - good sensitivity, good specificity
- for screening

Western blot: - extremely specific
- to confirm a positive ELISA

Antibodies are not detectable for 2-4 weeks after infection.

Part D : Fungi & Parasites

2.31.) FUNGI

WHAT THEY LOOK LIKE:

- Fungi come it two forms: **yeasts** (=single cells) and **molds** (=forming hyphae)

- Most fungi can be both (i.e. are dimorphic). Typically they form yeasts at 37°C and molds if they grow outside the human body.

EXAMPLES:

MOLDS	DIMORPHIC FUNGI	YEASTS
aspergillus • farmer's lung	**histoplasma** • pulmonary infection	**candida** • thrush, vaginitis
	blastomyces • respiratory tract infection	**cryptococcus** • pneumonia, meningitis
	coccidioides • desert rheumatism	

MOLDS:

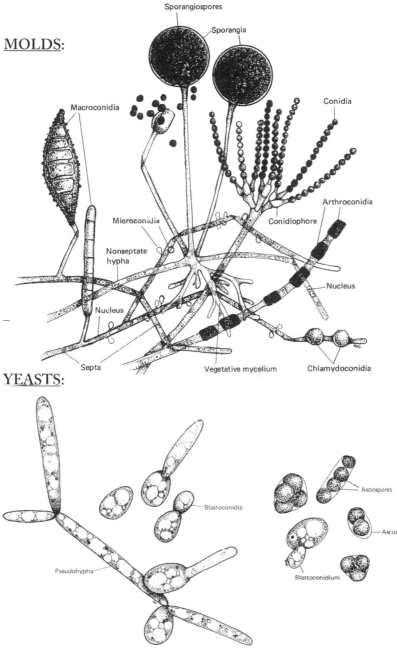

YEASTS:

From *Sherris Medical Microbiology*, 3rd edition, p. 574, edited by Kenneth J. Ryan.
Copyright 1994 by Appleton&Lange, Norwalk, Connecticut. Used with permission.

139

HOW THEY REPRODUCE:

- Fungi reproduce in two manners : Sexual and asexual.
- Most fungi can do both (i.e. *fungi perfecti*).
- Fungi that do not reproduce sexually are called *fungi imperfecti*.
  (or maybe they "couple" so rarely, that their spores went undetected so far…)

- **Sexual reproduction:** 2 cells fuse, diploid cell divides by meiosis
- **Asexual reproduction:** haploid cell divides by mitosis (like bacteria)

---

spores (sexual): Ascospores, Basidiospores, Zygospores etc.
conidia (asexual): Arthroconidia, Chlamydioconidia etc.

 Note, that both yeasts and molds can produce spores and conidia:

	YEASTS	MOLDS
asexual	Blastoconidia (="buds") Pseudohyphae	Arthroconidia Chlamydioconidia
sexual	Ascospores	Basidiospores Zygospores

2.32.) FUNGAL DISEASES

Clinically, fungi most often cause skin disease, but some can cause systemic infections. Immunocompromised patients may develop opportunistic fungal disease. Diagnosis is made by light microscopy using 10% KOH, which dissolves tissue but not fungal walls:

		MICROSCOPIC FEATURES
cutaneous	• dermatophytosis (ringworm)	o hyphae
	• tinea versicolor	o hyphae
subcutaneous	• mycetoma	o "tree" shaped (sporangia)
	• sporotrichosis	o cigar shaped budding yeast
systemic	• coccidioidomycosis	o soil: arthrospores tissue: endospores
	• histoplasmosis	o yeasts in macrophages
	• blastomycosis	o broad based bud with double refractory walls
opportunistic	• cryptococcosis	o capsule on India ink prep.
	• candidiasis	o pseudohyphae germ tubes
	• aspergillosis	o V shaped

Histoplasmosis: - humid soil (Mississippi river)
- most infections are asymptomatic
- progressive pulmonary disease resembles tuberculosis

Coccidioidomycosis: - "valley fever": fever, cough, arthralgia
- endemic to Arizona, Nevada, New Mexico.

Aspergillosis: - allergy, exacerbates asthma
- pulmonary disease (immunocompromised patients)
- radiologically visible fungus ball within cavity

2.33.) __MALARIA__

Malaria is found in most tropical areas and more than 1 million children die of the disease each year. Sporozoa are unique intracellular protozoa that cycle through sexual and asexual places of reproduction:

> **Mosquito: sexual cycle** → forms sporozoites
> **Human:**   **asexual cycle** → forms schizonts

1.)   **Sporozoites** are introduced into blood
2.)   Exo-erythrocytic phase: sporozoites differentiate into merozoites
3.)   **Merozoites** settle in liver (latent forms called hypnozoites)
4.)   Liver releases merozoites
5.)   Merozoites infect red blood cells
6.)   Ring-shaped **trophozoite** matures, forms multinucleated schizonts
7.)   RBC releases either 10-20 new merozoites or **gametocytes**

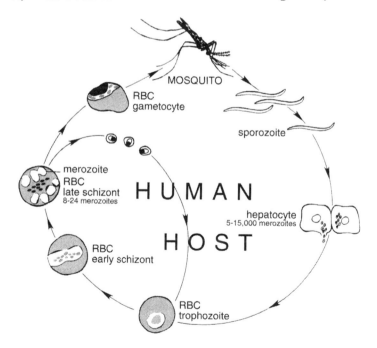

From *Sherris Medical Microbiology*, 3rd edition, p. 644, edited by Kenneth J. Ryan.
Copyright 1994 by Appleton&Lange, Norwalk, Connecticut. Used with permission.

Sporozoites reproduce asexually inside RBCs. Eventually the RBCs burst, causing periodic fever and anemia in the patient.

	KEY FEATURES
Vivax	• fever peak every 48 h • latent liver forms • very common
Ovale	• fever peak every 48 h • latent liver forms • rare
Falciparum	• fever peak every 48 h • most severe, life threatening • no trophozoites/schizonts found in blood • banana shaped gametocytes
Malariae	• fever peak every 72 h

<u>Prevention:</u>
1. mosquito screens, repellents
2. mefloquine or doxycycline when traveling to areas where chloroquine-resistance is common.

2.34.) TISSUE PROTOZOA

A) LATENT INFECTION IN MOST PEOPLE:

Pneumocystis jirovecii (~Pneumocystis carinii)	• it's a fungus, (but antifungal drugs are ineffective) • common in **AIDS** patients • sudden onset fever, dyspnea, tachypnea ➤ *TX: trimethoprim-sulfamethoxazole* *pentamidine*
Toxoplasma gondii	• natural host: GI tract of cats • cat feces, undercooked meat (pork) • cysts → invade gut wall → muscles, brain • severe **congenital defects** if pregnant woman gets infected ➤ *TX: sulfonamide (first trimester)* *sulfonamide-pyrimethamine (all others)*

B) TROPICAL/SUBTROPICAL: (transmitted by insects)

Leishmania	
a) L. donovani	**a)** Kala-Azar (visceral) "black sickness" (GI bleeding)
b) L. brasiliensis	**b)** Espundia (mucocutaneous ulcers)
c) L. mexicana, L. tropica	**c)** cutaneous leishmaniosis (red papule, satellites, ulcerating) ➤ *TX: sodium stibogluconate*
Trypanosoma	
a) T. cruzi (America)	**a)** kissing bug: **Chagas disease** ➤ *TX: nifurtimox*
b) T. gambiense (Africa)	**b)** Tsetse fly: **sleeping sickness**
c) T. rhodesiense (Africa)	**c)** more severe than T. gambiense ➤ *TX: suramin, melarsoprol*

2.35.) INTESTINAL PROTOZOA

Protozoa cause bloody diarrhea if they invade the wall of the GI tract. If they don't invade, the stool will be non-bloody. Interference with fat absorption results in greasy, foul-smelling stools that may float on water.

Entamoeba histolytica	• cysts have 4 nuclei • trophozoite: 1 nucleus, ingests red blood cells • bloody, mucus, diarrhea • liver abscess • can be sexually transmitted ➤ *TX: metronidazole*
Giardia lamblia (most common)	• cysts have 4 nuclei • trophozoite: 2 nuclei, 4 pairs of flagella (looks like a sad clown....) • excystation in duodenum • non-bloody, foul smelling diarrhea ➤ *TX: metronidazole*
Cryptosporidium	• excystation in small intestine • trophozoites do not invade gut wall • severe diarrhea in immunocompromised (AIDS!) patients ➤ *no effective therapy*

Compare trophozoite and cyst forms:

Entamoeba histolytica   Giardia lamblia

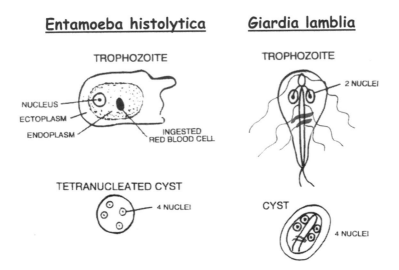

Modified from Gladwin and Trattler: *Clinical Microbiology Made Ridiculously Simple*, MedMaster, 2008

2.36.) TRICHOMONAS
very common sexually transmitted disease

Trichomonas

- 1 nucleus, 4 flagella, undulating membrane

- male: asymptomatic or non-purulent urethritis
- female: foul-smelling, watery, green discharge

➤ *TX: metronidazole*

2.37.) FLUKES
(Trematodes)

A) BLOOD FLUKES: (Schistosoma)

Intermediate host is a snail that releases larvae (*cercariae*) which can penetrate human skin. They enter small veins, pass through the right heart and lungs into the systemic circulation. After passing through intestinal capillaries, they settle in the portal vein where they mature to sexually active adults.

	ROUTE OF INFECTION:	EVENTUALLY SETTLES IN:
Sch. mansoni	penetrates skin	veins of colon
Sch. japonicum	penetrates skin	veins of small intestine
Sch. hematobium	penetrates skin	veins of urinary bladder

B) TISSUE FLUKES: (endemic to South East Asia)

	ROUTE OF INFECTION:	EVENTUALLY SETTLES IN:
Clonorchis sinensis	eating raw fish	**liver** → bile stones → bile obstruction → bile duct carcinoma
Paragonimus	eating raw crab meat	**lung** → eosinophilic inflammation

 Praziquantel eliminates flukes.

2.38.) TAPEWORMS
(Cestodes)

Long, ribbonlike worms that are the largest and most repulsive of intestinal parasites. If the patient ingested larvae, he becomes the primary host and the worms remain in the lumen of the gut. If the patient ingested eggs, he becomes an intermediate host: developing larvae invade the tissues and cause serious disease.

	SOURCE	INGESTED FORM	EVENTUALLY SETTLES IN:
T. solium [1]	pork	larvae	intestine
T. solium	human feces	eggs	brain, eyes (cysticerci)
T. saginata [2]	beef	larvae	intestine
D. latum	raw fish	larvae	intestine
Echinococcus	dog feces	eggs	in liver, lung, brain (cysts)

[1] *max. length: 5m* [2] *max. length: 10m*

Niclosamide eliminates tapeworms.

The tapeworm is long and flat and consists of a chain of box-like segments called **proglottids**. The head has suckers and sometimes hooks. maturation of the worm occurs from the anterior to the posterior end where fresh eggs are released.

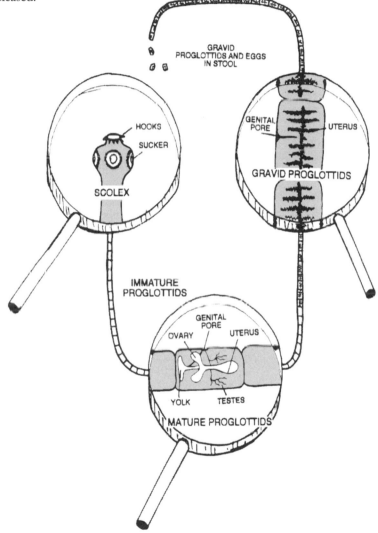

GRAVID PROGLOTTIDS AND EGGS IN STOOL

HOOKS

SUCKER

SCOLEX

GENITAL PORE

UTERUS

GRAVID PROGLOTTIDS

IMMATURE PROGLOTTIDS

GENITAL PORE

OVARY

UTERUS

YOLK

TESTES

MATURE PROGLOTTIDS

From Gladwin and Trattler: *Clinical Microbiology Made Ridiculously Simple*, MedMaster, 2008

2.39.) ROUNDWORMS
(Nematodes)

Intestinal nematodes are found in soil where human feces are deposited or used as fertilizer. Severity of disease depends on worm load and tissue invasion.

A) INGESTED FORM: EGGS

Enterobius	perianal pruritus (at night)
Ascaris	worm lives in colon, larvae migrate to lung

B) INGESTED FORM: LARVAE

Necator	intestinal blood loss
Strongyloides	larvae penetrate skin, then migrate to lung
Trichinella	pork meat, larvae form cysts in striated muscle

C) TRANSMITTED BY INSECT BITE:

Wuchereria	microfilariae found in blood adult worm lives in lymph nodes → lymph obstruction
Onchocerca	"river blindness" microfilariae in subcutaneous tissue and eye

Mebendazole and pyrantel pamoate eliminate roundworms.

PHARMACOLOGY

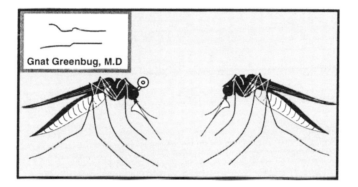

"Chemotherapy will increase your lifespan about 10 minutes, Mr. Mosley, which is not bad, given your normal life cycle of 2 days."

3.1.) DRUG INTERACTIONS

Drug to drug interactions account for a significant number of adverse reactions. They can diminish or potentiate the desired effects, which is most serious for drugs with a low therapeutic index (sulfonylureas, tolbutamide). Interactions may involve absorption, distribution, metabolism and excretion of drugs or may be due to direct competition near the receptor site.

drugs that become problematic when displaced from albumins	• sulfonamides • phenylbutazone • tolbutamide • coumarin
drugs that induce P450	• alcohol [1] • barbiturates • phenytoin • rifampicin
drugs that inhibit P450	• chloramphenicol • sulfonamides • phenylbutazone
drugs that compete for renal transporters	○ uric acid • probenecid • penicillins • sulfonamides • salicylates • thiazides

[1] *alcohol tolerance in heavy drinkers!*

EXAMPLES:

(1) Risk of severe hemorrhage if coumarins are combined with any other drug that competes for albumin.

(2) Sulfonamides displace sulfonylureas from albumin → hypoglycemia

(3) Barbiturate induces P450 enzyme → enhanced metabolism of MAO inhibitors → ineffective treatment of depression.

(4) P450 induction → Enhanced estrogen metabolism → reduced oral contraceptive efficacy → unplanned pregnancy

(5) Steroids compete with MAO inhibitor for P450 enzyme → reduced metabolism of MAO inhibitor → risk of over dose

(6) Aspirin reduces renal secretion of uric acid and is contraindicated in gout.

3.2.) BAD COMBINATIONS

NEVER EVER COMBINE:	WITH THESE DRUGS:
aminoglycosides	• neuromuscular blockers (enhanced block) • loop diuretics (compounds ototoxicity)
MAO inhibitors	• levodopa (hypertensive crisis) • amphetamine (hypertensive crisis) • tricyclic antidepressants [1]
tricyclic antidepressants	• MAO inhibitors [1]

[1] *antidepressants should never be combined with each other!*

3.3.) <u>FAMOUS SIDE EFFECTS</u>

There are at least as many questions on the USMLE about side effects of drugs as there are about main effects and mechanisms of action. Please study these very carefully!

FAMOUS SIDE EFFECT:	CAUSED BY:
anaphylactic shock	• penicillin • foreign proteins
hepatotoxicity	• isoniazid • halothane
renal toxicity	• phenacetin • other NSAIDs • cyclosporin
ototoxicity	• aminoglycosides
drug-induced lupus	• procainamide • hydralazine
photosensitivity (skin)	• tetracyclines • sulfonamides • sulfonylureas
cutaneous flushing	• niacin
hemolysis in patients with G6PD-deficiency	• sulfonamides • primaquine
bone marrow suppression	• chloramphenicol • ganciclovir • zidovudine (AZT)

3.4.) ANTIDOTES

Antitoxins are antibodies against bacterial toxins.
Antidotes interfere with the action or metabolism of toxic substances.

INTOXICATION BY	ANTIDOTE
acetaminophen	N-acetylcysteine
opiates	naloxone
benzodiazepines	flumazenil
methanol, ethylene glycol	ethanol
CO	100% O_2
cyanide	amyl nitrate
organophosphates	atropine, pralidoxime
iron	deferoxamine
lead	EDTA
coumarins	Vit. K
heparin	protamine

Intoxication with acidic drugs (e.g. barbiturate, salicylate):
Alkalinize urine (IV sodium-bicarbonate) to enhance renal excretion.

3.5.) <u>ANTIBIOTICS</u>

Bactericidal drugs "kill" bacteria.
Bacteriostatic drugs inhibit bacterial growth and require the
host's immune system to "finish the job".

BACTERICIDAL	BACTERIOSTATIC
• penicillins	• chloramphenicol
• cephalosporins	• erythromycin
• aminoglycosides	• tetracyclines
• vancomycin	• sulfonamides
• quinolones	• trimethoprim

*Misuse of antibiotics results in emergence of antibiotic-resistant
strains. This creates an ever-increasing need for new drugs…*

GRAM-POSITIVE	GRAM-NEGATIVE	BROAD-SPECTRUM
• penicillin G	• aminoglycosides	• ampicillin
• vancomycin	• polymyxins	• cephalosporins
• bacitracin		• tetracyclines
		• chloramphenicol
		• sulfonamides

MECHANISMS OF RESISTANCE

Bacteria become resistant to antibiotics if they acquire DNA coding for extra
enzymes (e.g. β-lactamase). There are 3 ways in which DNA may be acquired:

transduction	transmission of DNA by bacteriophages that carry plasmids (extrachromosomal DNA)
transformation	uptake and incorporation of DNA from environment
conjugation	direct transmission of DNA from cell to cell through the sex pilus

3.6.) <u>DRUGS OF CHOICE</u>

Actinomyces	actinomycosis	penicillin G
Bacillus anthracis	anthrax	ciprofloxacin, tetracyclines
Bordetella pertussis	whooping cough	erythromycin
Borrelia Burgdorferi	Lyme disease	tetracycline
Campylobacter	acute inflammatory diarrhea	ciprofloxacin
Candida	vaginal candidiasis	miconazole
	systemic candidiasis	fluconazole
Chlamydia trachomatis	pelvic inflammatory disease	doxycycline
Chlamydia pneumoniae	pneumonia	tetracycline
H. influenza	pneumonia, meningitis	3rd gen. cephalosporin
Helicobacter pylori	gastric ulcer	metronidazole + tetracycline
Klebsiella	pneumonia	3rd gen. cephalosporin
	UTI	quinolones
Legionella	Legionnaire's disease	erythromycin
M. tuberculosis	tuberculosis	isoniazid + rifampin
		+ pyrazinamide + ethambutol
M. leprae	leprosy	dapsone + rifampin
M. pneumoniae	atypical pneumonia	erythromycin
N. gonorrhea	gonorrhea	ceftriaxone
N. meningitis	meningitis	penicillin G
Nocardia	pneumonia	trimethoprim/sulfamethoxazole
Proteus	UTI	quinolones
Rickettsia	spotted fever, end. typhus	tetracycline
Salmonella typhi	typhoid fever	trimethoprim/sulfamethoxazole
Shigella	dysentery	trimethoprim/sulfamethoxazole
Staph. aureus	skin infection	dicloxacillin
	sepsis, osteomyelitis	nafcillin or oxacillin
Strept. pyogenes	pharyngitis, erysipelas	penicillin G or V
Strept. viridans	endocarditis	penicillin + aminoglycoside
Treponema pallidum	syphilis	penicillin G
Trichomonas	trichomoniasis	metronidazole
Tropheryma whippelii	Whipple's disease	trimethoprim/sulfamethoxazole
Vibrio cholerae	cholera	tetracycline (+ fluids!)
Yersinia pestis	plague ("black death")	streptomycin

3.7.) PENICILLINS

Penicillin G is the drug of choice for *Streptococci* and non-penicillinase producing *Staphylococci*. Broad spectrum penicillins are similar to Pen. G but are also effective against some gram- bacteria. Extended spectrum penicillins are for *Pseudomonas*, but lose their effectiveness against gram+ bacteria.

narrow spectrum β-lactamase sensitive	penicillin G penicillin V	gram positive *Strept.*
β-lactamase resistant	methicillin oxacillin nafcillin cloxacillin	gram positive *Strept.*
broad spectrum	ampicillin amoxicillin	*Hemophilus Neisseria E. coli Proteus*
extended spectrum	carbenicillin	*Pseudomonas*

☹

SIDE-EFFECTS
• allergic reactions (maculopapular rash, shock)
• cross-reactivity with cephalosporins
• diarrhea (disruption of normal GI flora)

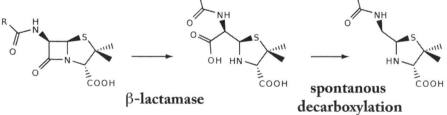

β-lactamase   spontanous decarboxylation

3.8.) <u>CEPHALOSPORINS</u>

Cephalosporins were developed as penicillin alternative. They are relatively safe and the newer generations have a broader spectrum against gram- bacteria.

<u>1st Generation</u> (against gram+ and *E. coli* and *Klebsiella*)

cefazolin	longest half life
cephalexin	acid stable (oral administration)

<u>2nd Generation</u> (broader spectrum against gram- bacilli)

cefamandole	⊗ disulfiram like reaction with ethanol bleeding (anti vitamin K action)
cefoxitin	potent against anaerobes (bowel perforation → *E. coli*, *Bacteroides fragilis*)

<u>3rd Generation</u> (superior activity against enterobacteriaceae)

cefotaxime	CNS permeable (*Hemophilus* meningitis!)
ceftriaxone	drug of choice for penicillin resistant gonorrhea

☹ | **SIDE-EFFECTS**
Avoid in patients with known penicillin allergy.
penicillin allergy.
(significant cross reactivity)

3.9.) ANTIVIRAL DRUGS

Many of the antiviral drugs resemble nucleosides and take advantage of differences between eukaryotic DNA-polymerase and viral polymerases. Other drugs inhibit viral enzymes needed for assembly.

	MECHANISM OF ACTION	USED TO TREAT
amantadine	impairs uncoating	influenza A
interferons	inhibits viral multiplication	leukemia Kaposi sarcoma genital warts hepatitis B and C
ribavirin	guanosine analog	RSV infections in children
acyclovir	guanine analog, depends on viral thymidine kinase	HSV-1, HSV-2, VZV
vidarabine	adenosine analog	all Herpes group viruses
idoxuridine	thymidine analog	Herpes simplex keratitis
ganciclovir	like acyclovir	CMV
AZT	thymidine analog	HIV
protease inhibitors	inhibit cleavage of the gag-pol polyprotein → noninfectious virus particles	HIV

AZT: 3'-azido-3'-deoxythymidine

3.10.) ANTIFUNGAL DRUGS

Most antifungal drugs interact with sterols in the fungus cell membrane, forming large pores. They are quite toxic and side-effects are common.

imidazoles	• broad spectrum anti-fungals • itraconazole and fluconazole have replaced the more toxic ketoconazole
amphotericin B, itraconazole	• for severe systemic fungal infections
nystatin powder	• candida skin infections
griseofulvin	• given orally but accumulates in keratin • dermatophytic Infections

☹

SIDE-EFFECTS

Griseofulvin: hepatotoxic, teratogenic
Amphotericin: nephrotoxic, anemia
Nystatin, miconazole: systemic toxicity
                                    (use only topically)

3.11.) ANTI-PROTOZOAL DRUGS

A) MALARIA:

Treatment of malaria requires destruction of (1.) erythrocyte schizont, (2.) erythrocyte gamete and (3.) liver schizont to prevent relapse.

prophylaxis	mefloquine or doxycycline
therapy	chloroquine
therapy *P. falciparum* [1]	mefloquine
prevention of relapse	primaquine [2]

[1] *usually resistant to chloroquine*
[2] *eradicates liver schizont of P. vivax and P. ovale*

B) OTHER PROTOZOA:

Amebiasis (*Trichomonas, Chlamydia*)	metronidazole
Leishmaniasis	stibogluconate
African sleeping sickness (*Trypanosoma gambiense*) (*Trypanosoma rhodesiense*)	melarsoprol / suramin
Chagas disease (*Trypanosoma cruzi*)	nifurtimox

3.12.) AIDS

A) TREATMENT OF HIV:

Combination of 2 to 4 drugs has become standard. This decreases the
likelihood of emergence of drug-resistant viral mutants.

		SIDE-EFFECTS
nucleosides	inhibit reverse transcriptase: • zidovudine (AZT) • didanosine (ddI)	• anemia, leukopenia • pancreatitis
non-nucleosides	inhibit reverse transcriptase: • Nevirapine (NVP)	• rashes
protease inhibitors	• Saquinavir (SAQ) • Indinavir (IND)	• kidney stones

B) TREATMENT OF OPPORTUNISTIC INFECTIONS:

Herpes simplex or zoster	acyclovir
CMV	ganciclovir
M. avium complex	clarithromycin + ethambutol
Candida (esophageal)	fluconazole, amphotericin B
Cryptococcus neoformans	fluconazole, amphotericin B
Pneumocystis carinii [1]	trimethoprim-sulfamethoxazole (pentamidine if allergic)
Toxoplasma gondii	pyrimethamine-sulfadiazine

[1] *prophylaxis necessary if CD4 < 200/µL*

3.13.) INHIBITORS OF TRANSLATION

RNA → Protein

A) PROKARYOTES:

Antibiotics which act on prokaryotic ribosomes (30S or 50S subunit):

	TARGET	MECHANISM OF ACTION
erythromycin	50 S	inhibits translocation
chloramphenicol	50 S	inhibits peptidyl transferase
aminoglycosides	30 S	inhibits initiation (binding of $tRNA_{fm}$)
tetracyclines	30 S	inhibits binding of all other tRNAs

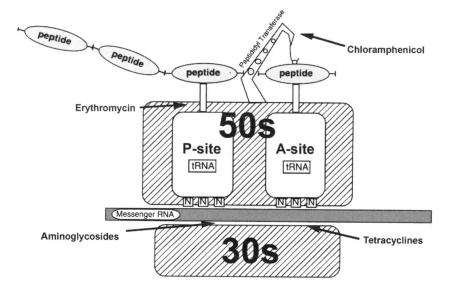

Modified from Olson: *Clinical Pharmacology Made Ridiculously Simple*, MedMaster, 2006

B) EUKARYOTES:

Chemicals that act on eukaryotic ribosomes (40S and 60S) are toxic and have no clinical use:

	TARGET	MECHANISM OF ACTION
lectins	40/60 S	inhibits initiation
cycloheximide	60 S	inhibits peptidyl transferase
dlphtheria toxin	60 S	inhibits elongation factor

B) PRO- AND EUKARYOTES:

	TARGET	MECHANISM OF ACTION
puromycin		incorporated into peptide chain → premature chain termination

3.14.) <u>INHIBITORS OF REPLICATION</u>
DNA → DNA

Most of these drugs interfere with replication of eukaryotic cells and are used for cancer treatment:

A) <u>ANTI-FOLATES</u>:

	MECHANISM OF ACTION	CLINICAL USE
methotrexate	mammalian folate synthesis	anticancer drug
trimethoprim	bacterial folate synthesis	antibiotic
pyrimethamine	protozoal folate synthesis	antimalarial

B) <u>PURINE ANALOGS</u>:

6-mercaptopurine	inhibits de novo synthesis	---
azathioprine	derivative of mercaptopurine	immunosuppressant

C) <u>PYRIMIDINE ANALOGS</u>:

cytarabine (ara-CTP)	incorporated into DNA	anticancer drug
5-fluorouracil	inhibits thymidylate synthesis	anticancer drug

D) <u>ANTIBIOTIC CYTOTOXINS</u>:

actinomycin D	binds to DNA	anticancer drug
doxorubicin	intercalates between base pairs	anticancer drug
bleomycin	causes strand breaks in DNA	anticancer drug

3.15.) <u>INHIBITORS OF TRANSCRIPTION</u>

DNA $\rightarrow$ RNA

A) <u>PROKARYOTES</u>:

rifampin	• binds to bacterial DNA-dependent RNA polymerase • inhibits initiation of RNA synthesis • anti-tuberculosis

B) <u>EUKARYOTES</u>:

α-amanitin	• blocks eukaryotic polymerase II • mushroom poison
actinomycin D	• binds to DNA • Inhibits transcription (low concentration) • inhibits replication (high concentration) anticancer drug
doxorubicin	• intercalates between base pairs • inhibits translation and replication anticancer drug

3.16.) COMBINATION CHEMOTHERAPY

"FAMOUS COMBINATIONS":

ALL	prednisone vincristine
Wilms tumor	dactinomycin vincristine
Hodgkin's disease[1]	**A** adriamycin **B** bleomycin **V** vinblastine **D** dacarbazine

[1] *ABVD has replaced MOPP as standard therapy!*

☹ SPECIFIC SIDE EFFECTS:

doxorubicin	cardiotoxic
bleomycin	pulmonary fibrosis
cisplatin	renal toxicity
cyclophosphamide	hemorrhagic cystitis
vincristine	peripheral neuropathy
L-asparaginase	allergic reactions

CYCLE-SPECIFIC DRUGS
bleomycin, vinca alkaloids, antimetabolites

3.17.) NSAIDs

NSAIDs decrease prostaglandin synthesis by inhibiting the key enzyme cyclooxygenase (COX). COX-1 controls many prostaglandins under "normal" conditions while COX-2 is active during inflammation. Selective COX-2 inhibitors have fewer side-effects than traditional NSAIDs.

GENERAL USE NSAIDs:

	MECHANISM OF ACTION	KEY FEATURES
aspirin	• acetylates cyclooxygenase	• **analgesic**: 600 mg/d • **anti-inflammatory**: 4g/d ☺ may cause Reye's syndrome ☹ contraindicated in gout !
acetaminophen	• no anti-inflammatory action • prefers CNS cyclooxygenase	• drug of choice for children with viral infections
ibuprofen	• similar spectrum as aspirin	• fewer GI side-effects
phenylbutazone	• anti-inflammatory • weak analgesic/antipyretic	• used when others have failed ☹ may cause skin rash, GI upset
indomethacin	• more potent anti-inflammatory than aspirin	• for acute gout • for ankylosing spondylitis ☹ may cause GI upset, pancreatitis
celecoxib	• selective COX-2 inhibitor	• chronic pain (osteoarthritis) ☹ risk of thrombosis, stroke, MI…

Aspirin: Acetylation of platelet cyclooxygenase is irreversible!
- don't give within 1 week prior to surgery!
- don't give if patient has bleeding disorder
- be careful with heparin!

SALICYLATE INTOXICATION
mild: tinnitus, central hyperventilation
severe: respiratory plus metabolic acidosis

SLOW-ACTING DRUGS FOR RHEUMATOID ARTHRITIS:

Slow-acting drugs are not useful for acute attacks but improve the course of this chronic disease.

	MECHANISM OF ACTION	KEY FEATURES
gold	• suppresses macrophages	• add when regular NSAIDs fail to suppress inflammation ☹ dermatitis, aplastic anemia
D-penicillamine	• reduces rheumatoid factor	• when gold has failed or is too toxic ☹ bone marrow suppression
methotrexate[1]	• folic acid antagonist	• when all else has failed ☹ bone marrow suppression ☹ liver failure

[1] *much lower dose than what is used for cancer therapy.*

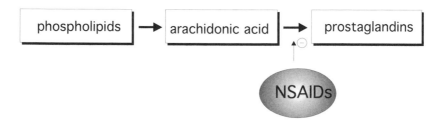

3.18.) *GOUT*

Acute or chronic arthritis that results from deposition of urate crystals in and around joints. Treatment of acute gout differs from that of chronic gout:

		MECHANISM OF ACTION
acute attack	**colchicine**	• inhibits migration of macrophages (depolymerizes microtubules) ☹ vomiting, abdominal pain
chronic gout	**allopurinol**	• purine analog • inhibits xanthine oxidase ☹ hypersensitivity reaction
chronic gout	**probenecid**	• blocks tubular secretion of penicillin [1] • blocks tubular reabsorption of uric acid

[1] *occasionally used to increase serum levels of antibiotics.*

CAUSES OF CHRONIC GOUT
• elevated uric acid
• Lesch–Nyhan syndrome
• treatment of malignancies

Most people with elevated uric acid levels do NOT have gout!

3.19.) <u>HEART FAILURE</u>

Sites of action for drugs used to treat heart failure: Drugs that work in the heart enhance myocardial contractility, whereas drugs that work on other sites reduce either PRELOAD or AFTERLOAD.

Diuretics do so by decreasing blood volume. Vasodilators increase the space provided for the blood, thus reducing pressure.

Angiotensin converting enzyme (ACE) inhibitors block the synthesis of the vasoconstrictor angiotensin-II in the lungs. This also reduces aldosterone secretion from the adrenals, leading to water loss and reduction in blood volume.

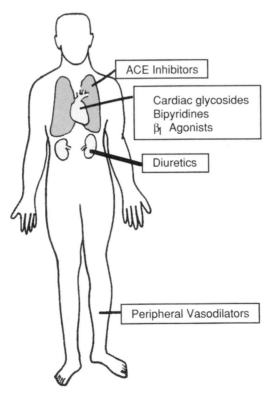

From Olson: *Clinical Pharmacology Made Ridiculously Simple*, MedMaster, 1994

3.20.) ANTIHYPERTENSIVE DRUGS

Before treating a patient with "essential" hypertension, rule out specific causes: (1.) renal diseases, (2.) aldosteronism, (3.) coarctation of aorta, (4.) pheochromocytoma. Choice of drug depends on clinical setting and contraindications:

	CLINICAL SETTING	CONTRAINDICATIONS
Ca^{2+} channel blockers	• for all patients	• CHF
β-blockers	• angina pectoris • post MI	• diabetes • asthma • peripheral vascular disease
thiazides	• CHF • chronic renal failure	• diabetes • hyperlipidemia
ACE inhibitors	• for all patients	• pregnancy

CHF = congestive heart failure

Hypertensive crisis*: -sodium nitroprusside is rapid and potent.*
                              - use only in hospital-setting.

SIDE-EFFECTS
β-blockers: - depression, fatigue, lethargy
             - increased plasma triglycerides
thiazides: - hypokalemia
             - hypercalcemia

173

3.21.) ANTI-ANGIOTENSINS

Renin converts angiotensinogen to Ang-I. Angiotensin converting enzyme (ACE) converts Ang-I to the biologically active Ang-II which acts on angiotensin receptors on smooth muscle as a very potent vasoconstrictor.

	KEY FEATURES
captopril	• ACE inhibitor • decreases angiotensin II • increases bradykinin
enalapril	• ACE inhibitor • more potent • longer half time
saralasin	• blocks angiotensin receptors (weak agonist)

ACE inhibitors work particularly well in young, white patients.

3.22.) ERGOT ALKALOIDS

Ergot is a product of a fungus growing on rye and other grains.

	MECHANISM OF ACTION	INDICATIONS
ergotamine, methysergide	vasoconstriction	• to abort migraine attack • post partum hemorrhage (contracts uterus)
bromocriptine	inhibits prolactin release	• hyperprolactinemia (pituitary adenomas) • infertility

☹ *diarrhea, nausea, severe vasospasms*

174

3.23.) DIURETICS

Diuretics increase the rate of urine formation. More important than just the volume of urine is the net loss of solute which mobilizes edema fluid. Diuretics are classified by the site of their action on renal tubules:

		INDICATIONS	® SIDE EFFECTS
carb. anhydrase inhibitors	acetazolamide	• weak diuretic • rarely used	• metabolic acidosis [1]
loop diuretics	furosemide, ethacrynic acid	• acute pulmonary edema • hypercalcemia	• ototoxicity • hypokalemia • hyperuricemia
thiazides	chlorothiazide, hydrochlorothiazide, chlorthalidone	• hypertension • mild congestive heart failure • urinary calcium stones • diabetes insipidus	• hypokalemia • hypercalcemia • hyperglycemia • hyperuricemia
potassium sparing	spironolactone, (aldosterone antagonist) amiloride, triamterene	• usually combined with thiazides or loop diuretics • secondary hyperaldosteronism	• gynecomastia • menstrual irregularity
osmotic diuretics	mannitol	• acute renal failure • not useful in conditions a/w Na^+ retention	

[1] *useful to prevent "mountain sickness" (respiratory alkalosis).*

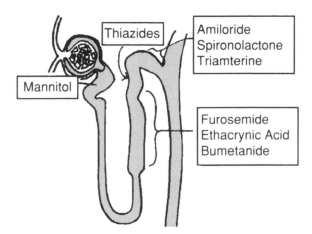

3.24.) <u>ANTIANGINAL DRUGS</u>

Angina pectoris occurs when cardiac work and O_2 demand exceed the ability of coronary arteries to supply oxygenated blood. Antianginal drugs relax smooth muscles and are potent vasodilators.

	KEY FEATURES
nitroglycerin	• low dose : dilates veins, reduces preload • high dose: also dilates arterioles, reflex tachycardia (angina may get worse)
Isosorbide dinitrate	• orally active • less potent than nitroglycerin
nifedipine	• relaxes arterioles • best for Prinzmetal's angina (coronary artery spasm)
verapamil	• slows heart rate • effect partially overcome by reflex tachycardia

Nitroglycerin generates metHb (Fe^{3+}) which can bind toxic cyanide – very useful as antidote!

3.25.) <u>PLATELET AGGREGATION INHIBITORS</u>

Whether platelets aggregate or not depends on the balance of inhibitors (PGI_2) and activators (thromboxane A_2) acting on surface receptors. Activated platelets release serotonin, ADP and additional thromboxane A_2.

	MECHANISM OF ACTION
aspirin	• inhibits cyclooxygenase (blocks thromboxane A_2 synthesis)
sulfinpyrazone	• inhibits degranulation (serotonin, ADP) • prolongs platelet survival
dipyridamole	• phosphodiesterase inhibitor • increases cAMP → inhibits degranulation

---

Prostacyclin → increases platelet cAMP → inhibits degranulation
Thromboxane A_2 → activates platelets (IP_3, DAG) → degranulation

Platelets release ADP and thromboxane A_2 → activate other platelets

---

Used for:
- *prophylaxis of transient ischemic attacks*
- *decrease mortality in postmyocardial patients*

3.26.) ANTICOAGULANTS

Patients with deep vein thrombosis are first placed on heparin (injectable, fast acting) to prevent pulmonary embolism. Coumarins are taken orally and anticoagulant effect develops slowly.

	MECHANISM OF ACTION	ANTAGONIST
heparin	• enhances activity of antithrombin III	protamine sulfate
warfarin dicumarol	• antagonist of vit. K (II, VII, IX, X)	vitamin K

> **Monitor therapy with anticoagulants:**
> Warfarin: prothrombin time (PT) **or INR**: extrinsic pathway
> Heparin: partial thromboplastin time (aPPT): intrinsic pathway

3.27.) THROMBOLYTICS

Thrombolytic drugs are used to dissolve blood clots (acute MI)

	MECHANISM OF ACTION	ANTAGONIST
streptokinase	• derived from streptococci • activates plasminogen (plasmin then degrades fibrin)	aminocaproic acid
urokinase	• derived from human fetal renal cells • less antigenicity than streptokinase	
TPA	• "fibrin selective" [1]	

[1] *activates only plasminogen already bound to fibrin*

3.28.) <u>ANTIARRHYTHMIC DRUGS</u>

All antiarrhythmic drugs have the potential to induce arrhythmias. Therapy sometimes is a matter of "trial and error". These drugs are classified by their action on the cardiac action potential:

class 1	Na^+ channel blockers
class 2	β-blockers
class 3	K^+ channel blockers
class 4	Ca^{2+} channel blockers

CLASS	DRUGS	APD	UV	INDICATIONS
1A	quinidine, procainamide	↑	↓	• ectopic arrhythmias
1B	lidocaine, phenytoin	↓	↓	• acute ventricular flutter/fibrillation • digitalis induced arrhythmias
1C	flecainide encalnide	∅	↓	• "broad spectrum" antiarrhythmic
2	propanolol			• atrial tachycardia • post MI (prophylactic)
3	bretylium amiodarone			• severe unresponsive ventricular arrhythmias
4	verapamil			• atrial tachycardia • atrial flutter

ADP: *Action potential duration*   **UV:** *Upstroke velocity*

☹
SIDE-EFFECTS	
procainamide:	reversible lupus erythematosus
phenytoin:	gingiva hyperplasia
quinidine:	potentiates digitoxin toxicity

3.29.) INOTROPIC DRUGS

increased strength of cardiac contractions → increased stroke volume

Cardiac glycosides derived from the foxglove plant inhibit Na^+/K^+ ATPase. Increased intracellular Na^+ levels decrease Na^+/Ca^{2+} exchanger, resulting in elevated Ca^{2+} and stronger muscle contraction (positive inotropic effect).

		KEY FEATURES
glycosides	digoxin, digitoxin	• glycosides have a low therapeutic index! • digoxin: short, digitoxin: long action
β-agonists	dobutamine, dopamine	• β-agonists increase cAMP • less tachycardia or peripheral side effects than isoproterenol or epinephrine
PDE inhibitors	amrinone	☹ thrombocytopenia
	milrinone	☺ does not affect platelets

Dopamine enhances renal blood flow and is particularly useful for treatment of shock.

GLYCOSIDE SIDE-EFFECTS

extracardiac: - nausea, abdominal pain
- fatigue
- confusion, disorientation
- color misperception: yellow

cardiac: - AV block, arrhythmias

Toxicity of glycosides is enhanced by:
➤ hypokalemia
➤ alkalosis
➤ hypoxia
➤ hypothyroidism

3.30.) <u>ASTHMA</u>

Asthma is due to type I hypersensitivity reaction of the airways. Treatment aims at relaxing bronchial smooth muscles and reducing airway inflammation:

DRUG	INDICATION	MECHANISM OF ACTION
metaproterenol, terbutaline, albuterol	mild, intermittent asthma	β_2-selective agonists
theophylline	more severe asthma	phosphodiesterase inhibitor → cAMP ↑
cromolyn	prophylaxis	stabilizes mast cells
corticosteroids (inhaled)	severe, chronic asthma	anti-inflammatory
corticosteroids I.V.	status asthmaticus	anti-inflammatory

☹ SIDE-EFFECTS
β_2-agonists: - tremor
                  - dizziness, palpitations
theophylline: - arrhythmias, seizures

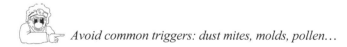 *Avoid common triggers: dust mites, molds, pollen…*

3.31.) INSULINS
for treatment of IDDM = type 1

Hyperglycemia is responsible for most of the long-term complications of diabetes. Therapy attempts to lower HbA$_{1C}$ (indicator of glucose during preceding 1-3 months) while avoiding hypoglycemic reactions.

		PEAK	DURATION
CZI	**"regular insulin"**	30 min	120 min
semilente	given subcutaneously rapid onset	2-3 h	5-8 h
lente	mix of semi and ultra	8-12 h	18-24 h
ultralente	prolonged action	14-20 h	36 h
PZI	CZI treated with protamine	24 h	36 h

Beef and pork insulin has been replaced in US by synthetic insulin, made by recombinant DNA technology in E.coli. The two protein chains (α and β) are harvested and combined in the laboratory.

☹

SIDE-EFFECTS
hypoglycemia: sweating, anxiety, tremor, weakness
fat atrophy: at site of injection

A common schedule:
- mix CZI and NPH (lente)
- give twice daily (morning and evening)
- monitor glucose in morning and afternoon

3.32.) <u>SULFONYLUREAS</u>
for treatment of NIDDM = type 2

Sulfonylureas lower plasma glucose by stimulating insulin secretion. They block K^+ channels of β-pancreatic cells, leading to membrane depolarization, increased intracellular Ca^{2+} and insulin secretion.

	DURATION OF ACTION
tolbutamide	8 h
glyburide, glipizide	20 h, most potent
chlorpropamide	48 h

Sulfonylureas are contraindicated in patients with liver or kidney failure: Accumulation will increase risk of hypoglycemia (especially with chlorpropamide)

Sulfonylureas are tightly bound to albumin. Competition with other albumin-binding drugs results in dangerous hypoglycemia.

3.33.) <u>HYPERLIPIDEMIAS</u>

Hyperlipidemia increases the risk of coronary artery disease – "good" cholesterol (HDL) lowers the risk, "bad" cholesterol (LDL) increase the risk. Here is how to calculate LDL from measurement of other blood lipids:

$$LDL = \text{Total Cholesterol} - HDL - (\text{Triglycerides} / 5)$$

<u>TYPES OF HYPERLIPIDEMIA:</u>

	ELEVATED FRACTION	DEFECT
Type I	chylomicrons *(triglycerides)*	lipoprotein lipase
Type IIA	LDL *(cholesterol)*	LDL receptor
Type IIB	LDL *(cholesterol)* VLDL *(triglycerides)*	mutant apoprotein ?
Type III	IDL *(triglycerides and cholesterol)*	mutant apoprotein E
Type IV	VLDL 1 *(triglycerides)*	overproduction of VLDL underutilization of VLDL

3.34.) HYPERLIPIDEMIA DRUGS

Diet is the most important factor, improving all types. Drugs are indicated for genetic causes, or if lipid levels cannot be controlled by diet alone.

	MECHANISM OF ACTION / SIDE-EFFECTS	INDICATION
diet	• helps all types of hyperlipidemia • is the only option for type I	**all types**
niacin	• inhibits lipolysis in fat cells • decreases free fatty acids (decreased VLDL synthesis) ☹ cutaneous flush	**type IIB**
clofibrate	• activates lipoprotein lipase (increases VLDL utilization) • inhibits cholesterol synthesis • enhances cholesterol excretion in bile ☹ forms gallstones	**types III, IV**
cholestyramine colestipol	• anion exchanger (binds cholesterol in gut) ☹ interferes with absorption of many drugs[1]	**types IIA, IIB**
lovastatin	• inhibits HMG-CoA reductase ☹ liver toxicity contraindicated during pregnancy	**types IIA, IIB**

[1] *don't give at same time of day!*

3.35.) PEPTIC ULCERS

H. pylori is the primary cause of peptic ulcer disease, rendering the mucosa susceptible to acids. Eradication of *H. pylori* usually leads to lasting remission.

H$_2$ blockers	**cimetidine**	☹ anti-androgenic action
	ranitidine	• more potent, longer acting • no anti-androgenic action
	famotidine	• most potent
prostaglandins	**misoprostol**	• analog of PGE
proton pump inhibitors	**omeprazole**	• **drug of choice !**
anti muscarinic	**pirenzepine**	• reduces acid secretion • less effect on motility • usually combined with others
antacids	**Al (OH)$_3$**	☹ may cause constipation
	Mg (OH)$_3$	☹ may cause diarrhea
mucosa protection	**bismuth sucralfate**	

> **Eradication of *H. pylori***
> metronidazole + tetracycline + bismuth

Refractory ulcers → suspect Zollinger-Ellison syndrome.
(gastrinoma of pancreas or duodenum)

3.36.) ADRENERGIC DRUGS

A) DIRECT ADRENERGIC DRUGS act directly on adrenergic receptors.

		RECEPTOR ACTION	MAIN INDICATIONS
α-blockers	• phenoxybenzamine • phentolamine • prazosin	α1 , α2, irreversible α1 , α2, reversible α1	• autonomic hyperreflexia • hypertensive crisis • hypertension
α-agonists	• phenylephrine • methoxamine • clonidine	α1 α1 α2 , central action	• nasal decongestant • hypotension • hypertension
β-blockers	• propanolol • pindolol • metoprolol • atenolol • labetalol	β1 , β2 β1 , β2 , intrinsic act. β1 β1 β , α	• hypertension • migraine prophylaxis • glaucoma
β-agonists	• isoproterenol • metaproterenol, albuterol, terbutaline • dobutamine • dopamine	β1 , β2 β2 β1 D1 > β1	• AV block • bronchospasm • congestive heart failure • shock

B) INDIRECT ADRENERGIC DRUGS modify the amount of norepinephrine at the postsynaptic membrane.

indirect -	• reserpine • guanethidine	depletes neuro- transmitter stores	• hypertension • hypertension
indirect +	• ephedrine • amphetamine	prolongs neuro- transmitter action	• nasal decongestant • narcolepsy, ADHD

3.37.) CHOLINESTERASE INHIBITORS

Acetylcholinesterase splits ACh into acetate and choline and terminates its action. Inhibitors of this enzyme increase the amount of ACh at the neuromuscular junction and parasympathetic nerve endings

	USE	KEY FEATURES
physostigmine	treatment of M.G.	☹ may cause CNS convulsions
neostigmine	treatment of M.G.	• does not enter CNS • better action on skeletal muscle
edrophonium	diagnosis of M.G.	• shortest duration of action
organophosphates	nerve gas insecticide	• irreversible (highly toxic)

M.G. = myasthenia gravis (autoantibodies against muscle ACh receptor)

Diagnosis of myasthenia gravis (Tensilon test)
Myasthenic crisis: edrophonium improves muscle strength
Cholinergic crisis: edrophonium further reduces muscle strength

Organophosphates directly inhibit ACh esterase and slowly form an irreversible complex with the esterase ("aging"). Pralidoxime prevents "aging" and releases active ACh esterase when given early.

3.38.) <u>CHOLINERGIC DRUGS</u>

<u>DIRECT MUSCARINIC DRUGS</u> stimulate muscarinic receptors at parasympathetic nerve terminals

	MAIN INDICATIONS	RECEPTOR ACTION
bethanechol	• atonic bladder	muscarinic
pilocarpine [1]	• acute glaucoma	muscarinic
carbachol [1]	• glaucoma • not hydrolyzed by ACh-esterase	muscarinic / nicotinic

[1] *produces miosis (small pupils*
opens outflow (canal of Schlemm) → *reduces ocular pressure*

 Automatic bladder: Spinal cord damage above sacral cord
→ *micturition reflex intact*
→ *conscious control over this reflex is lost*

Atonic bladder: Caused by destruction of sensory nerves
Injury to sacral spinal cord → *loss of micturition reflex*

Spinal shock: *temporary loss of micturition reflex*

3.39.) ANTI-MUSCARINIC DRUGS

➤ inhibit muscarinic receptors at parasympathetic nerve terminals

	USE
atropine	• anti-spasmodic • mydriasis (large pupils) to facilitate ophthalmologic examination • antidote for organophosphate poisoning
scopolamine	• greater CNS action than atropine for motion sickness

3.40.) ANTI-NICOTINIC DRUGS

➤ inhibit nicotinic receptors at the motor endplates

	ACTIONS / USE
tubocurarine	• blocks nicotinic ACh receptor • muscle relaxant (surgery) ☹ histamine release → bronchospasm hypotension
pancuronium	☺ less histamine release than tubocurarine
succinyl choline	• depolarizing • very short duration of action ☹ post-op muscle pain and stiffness risk of malignant hyperthermia [1]

[1] Ca^{2+} *release from SR* → *muscles generate heat* → *life threatening!*

Be careful with drugs that enhance neuromuscular block:
➤ halothane
➤ aminoglycosides
➤ Ca^{2+} channel blockers

3.41.) <u>ORAL CONTRACEPTIVES</u>

A) <u>USES</u>:

estrogen	• **"morning after pill"**
progesterone	• **"mini pill"** • habitual abortion • endometriosis
combination	• oral contraceptive • hormone replacement

B) <u>SIDE-EFFECTS</u>:

Oral contraceptives contain a mixture of estrogen and progesterone. You should adjust the prescription depending on the side effect your patient experiences:

ESTROGENS ☹	PROGESTERONES ☹
• nausea • vomiting • breast tenderness • skin pigmentation • hypertension • breakthrough bleeding	• weight gain • depression • hirsutism

---

RISKS OF ORAL CONTRACEPTIVES
- ➤ thromboembolia
- ➤ benign adenoma of the liver
- ➤ vaginal cancer in daughters of mothers who received DES

- ➤ <u>very slight</u> breast cancer or endometrial cancer
  (provided estrogen is combined with progesterone!)

3.42.) <u>STREET DRUGS</u>

<u>HALLUCINOGENS</u>:

	KEY FEATURES

LSD	• acts on 5-HT$_1$ and 5-HT$_2$ receptors
	
	• activates sympathetic system → arousal
	                                           tachycardia
	                                           sweating
	• brilliant color hallucinations
	  (these are blockable by neuroleptics)
	• may trigger schizophreniform psychosis
	• flashbacks

MDMA ("raves")	• popular at dance scene "the raves" • euphoria and confidence • deaths have occurred due to dehydration

 Flashback: *Recurrence of drug effect without the drug.*

<u>OTHERS</u>:

	KEY FEATURES
THC (marihuana)	• enhanced sensory activity • impaired mental activity, sleepiness • altered sense of time and self • impaired short term memory • red conjunctivas
phencyclidine ("angel dust")	• reuptake inhibitor • mood elevation, sense of intoxication • bizarre and aggressive behavior

(see 3.46 for amphetamines)

3.43.) OPIOIDS

Opioids have the potential to cause strong psychological and physical dependence. Withdrawal ($\rightarrow$CNS hyperactivity) is severe, but self-limited and not life-threatening.

A) ENDORPHINS (ENDOGENOUS OPIOID PEPTIDES):

	RECEPTOR	EFFECT
met-enkephalin	mu	• euphoria, dependence • analgesia • respiratory depression
leu-enkephalin	delta	• mood changes
dynorphin	kappa	• analgesia, miosis, sedation

 Morphine (like met-enkephalin) acts on mu receptors.

B) SYNTHETIC OPIOIDS:

Tend to be under-prescribed because of physicians' fear of causing dependence…

	KEY FEATURES
naloxone	• μ, κ, σ antagonist • reverses morphine overdose
pentazocine	• κ, σ agonist / δ, μ antagonist • less effective for severe pain than morphine • less potential for dependence
codeine	• weak analgesic ("as strong as aspirin") • good antitussive • low abuse potential
propoxyphene	**dextro:** analgesic **levo:** antitussive
fentanyl	• 80x analgesic potency of morphine
methadone	• longer duration of action than morphine • used for controlled withdrawal

3.44.) ANTIDEPRESSANTS

Response to antidepressants takes 3–4 weeks. Therapy should continue for several months.
Ask your patient about suicide and offer supportive (not analytic!) psychotherapy.

	MECHANISM OF ACTION	KEY FEATURES
"New Generation" fluoxetine trazodone	• selectively block **serotonin** (5-HT) uptake	• drug of first choice ☺ no anticholinergic side-effects 5-HT1 → antidepressant 5-HT2 → nervousness, insomnia 5 HT3 → nausea, headache
Tricyclic antidepressants amitriptyline amoxapine desipramine etc.	• block neurotransmitter uptake (NE, serotonin, dopamine) • block receptors (m, α, serotonin, histamine)	• slow onset of action • inconsistent bioavailability ☹ <u>**anticholinergic side-effects:**</u> - blurred vision, dry mouth - constipation - urinary retention
MAO inhibitors	• increases amount of transmitter stored	• use when other drugs have failed • have stimulant properties • caveat: tyramine

Tyramine (cheese, beer, red wine) normally is inactivated by MAO in gut.
When it gets into the circulation → hypertensive crisis!

3.45.) LITHIUM

Therapeutic range: 0.5-1 mEq/L

Lithium is a "mood-stabilizer", effective for bipolar disorder and isolated manic episodes. Treatment of a manic episode should continue for at least 6 months. Because of its very low therapeutic index you must carefully monitor your patients for side-effects:

key features	☹ extremely low therapeutic index • excreted by kidneys
indications	• to treat manic episodes • to stabilize mood (prevents both manic and depressive episodes)
"normal" side-effects	• mild nausea • thirst
early intoxication 1.5 - 2 mEq/L	• abdominal pain, vomiting • hand tremor • ataxia, nystagmus • slurred speech
severe intoxication > 2 mEq/L	• persistent vomiting • blurred vision • hyperactive tendon reflexes • convulsions, coma, death

3.46.) CNS STIMULANTS

CNS stimulants cause psychological dependence (most profound for cocaine). Physical dependence is less with these drugs.

	KEY FEATURES
methylxanthines caffeine, theophylline	**low dose:** increased alertness **high dose:** anxiety, tremors • smooth muscle relaxation • weak diuretic • enhanced acid secretion in stomach
nicotine	**low dose:** ganglion stimulating, BP ↑ **high dose:** ganglion blockade, BP ↓
cocaine	• reuptake inhibitor • local anesthetic and vasoconstrictor • euphoria, hallucinations delusions, paranoia • cardiac arrhythmias
crack cocaine	• quicker effect, more intense "high"
amphetamines	• release of stored catecholamines • effects like cocaine • euphoria lasts longer than cocaine • no tolerance to CNS toxicity
methamphetamines	• common form of amphetamine abuse in US • can be smoked as "ice"

Dextroamphetamine: *- strong appetite suppressant*
                      - euphoria, risk of dependence
                      - not recommended for weight loss!

3.47.) ANXIOLYTIC DRUGS

Anxiety is often a/w medical or psychiatric problems. Best response to anxiolytics occurs in relatively acute anxiety reactions. Chronic use may lead to dependence.

		KEY FEATURES
benzodiazepines	**diazepam**	• long acting • for status epilepticus
	chlordiazepoxide	• long acting • for alcohol withdrawal
	lorazepam, triazolam	• rapid elimination (short half life) > ☹ severe withdrawal symptoms
others	**buspirone**	• acts on 5-HT1A receptors • slow onset of action • less sedation • less dependence

Abrupt withdrawal may cause delirium and seizures!

3.48.) HYPNOTIC DRUGS

These drugs cause widespread depression of CNS → risk of respiratory depression
(suicidal potential)

		KEY FEATURES
barbiturates	**phenobarbital**	• long acting, for seizure disorder
	thiopental	• short acting, for anesthesia
others	**chloral hydrate**	• short term use for insomnia ☹ "date rape drug"
	meprobamate	• less sedation, better anxiolytic

3.49.) ANTIHISTAMINES

A) RECEPTORS:

H1 receptors	• nasal and bronchial secretions • constrict bronchial smooth muscle → asthma • dilate skin capillaries → redness, wheals, itch
H2 receptors	• acid secretion in stomach

B) RECEPTOR BLOCKERS:

Antihistamines are the drug of choice for allergic rhinitis and urticaria.
Their major side-effect is sedation:

	KEY FEATURES
diphenhydramine	indications: • allergic rhinitis • urticaria • not effective in asthma ☹ sedation
carbinoxamine	☺ less drowsiness than diphenhydramine
trimeprazine (phenothiazine)	• long half life • good antipruritic
terfenadine, astemizole	• non-sedating antihistamines

> ### For motion sickness and nausea
> • diphenhydramine (antihistamine)
> • meclizine (antihistamine)
> • scopolamine (phenothiazine)

3.50.) ANESTHETICS

The minimum alveolar concentration (MAC) is the gas concentration needed to prevent movement of patients subjected to painful stimuli. MAC depends on the blood/gas partition (solubility). If the partition coefficient is high, a low alveolar concentration is sufficient but onset and termination of anesthesia will be slow.

MAC :	N_2O > enflurane > halothane
onset :	N_2O > enflurane > halothane
	fastest......................slowest

A) INHALATION:

	KEY FEATURES
halothane	• lacks analgesic potency ☹ hepatotoxic for adults cardiac arrhythmias malignant hyperthermia
enflurane	• excreted by kidneys rather than liver
isoflurane	• does not induce arrhythmias • lower toxicity
N_2O (nitrous oxide)	• not potent • does not depress respiration • safe

B) I.V.:

thiopental	• ultrashort barbiturate • not analgesic
ketamine	• dissociative anesthesia (patient appears awake but is unaware of pain) ☹ postoperative hallucinations

> ➤ **Balanced anesthesia:** thiopental + fentanyl + tubocurarine + N_2O
> ➤ **Neurolept anesthesia:** droperidol + fentanyl + N_2O

3.51.) PARKINSON'S DISEASE

Parkinson's is due to loss of dopaminergic substantia nigra neurons which project to the basal ganglia. This results in a neurotransmitter imbalance. Symptoms can be improved by either increasing dopamine or decreasing acetylcholine in the basal ganglia:

dopaminergic	**levodopa**	• CNS permeable dopamine • (**carbidopa** inhibits periph. decarboxylase) ☹ nausea, vomiting dyskinesia psychic disturbances
	bromocriptine	• direct dopamine agonist
	deprenyl	• inhibits MAO-B (dopamine selective)
	amantadine	• enhances dopamine metabolism
anticholinergic	**benztropine** **biperiden**	☹ dry mouth mydriasis tachycardia constipation urinary retention

<u>Early disease:</u>
If symptoms are mild, no drugs may be necessary
Otherwise start with anticholinergics or amantadine

<u>Fully developed disease:</u>
Levodopa plus Carbidopa

<u>Late stage:</u>
"wearing off" of drug effect
"on-off" phenomenon
may need to reduce levodopa if dyskinesias develop
may need to combine several drugs

3.52.) NEUROLEPTICS

Antipsychotic drugs (neuroleptics) are used to treat schizophrenia. They have a high affinity for dopamine D2 receptors. Their Parkinson-like side effects are due to block of dopamine receptors in the basal ganglia.

		KEY FEATURES
phenothiazines	**chlorpromazine**	☹ anticholinergic side effects arrhythmias rarely used
	fluphenazine	• long acting • for outpatients
butyrophenones	**haloperidol**	☹ extrapyramidal side effects fewer anticholinergic side effects
	droperidol	• for neurolept anesthesia
other	**clozapine**	☹ bone marrow suppression fewer extrapyramidal side effects

---

☹ DYSKINESIAS CAUSED BY NEUROLEPTICS

- **Acute dystonia** occurs within hours of administration.
- torticollis, jaw dislocation, tongue protrusion
  usually disappears (tolerance)

- **Parkinsonism** occurs within weeks to months of treatment.
- muscle stiffness, cogwheel rigidity, shuffling, drooling
  usually disappears (tolerance)

- **Tardive dyskinesia** occurs after many months of treatment.
- choreoathetosis, tongue protrusion, lateral movements of jaw
  may be irreversible!

3.53.) ANTIEPILEPTIC DRUGS

Seizures are due to sudden abnormal electrical activity in the cortex. It may be focal or spread and cause generalized convulsions. Antiepileptic drugs reduce neuronal excitability and prolong the refractory period of the action potentials.

DISORDER	DRUG OF CHOICE
generalized tonic-clonic *(grand mal)*	phenytoin, carbamazepine
absence seizures *(petit mal)*	ethosuximide
partial focal	phenytoin, carbamazepine
myoclonic	valproic acid, clonazepam
febrile seizures (children)	phenobarbital
status epilepticus [1]	diazepam I.V.

[1] *Medical emergency! Keep airways open!*

3.54.) ANTIEMETIC DRUGS

Antiemetics act on the chemoreceptor trigger zone of the brain stem (vomiting center). For unknown reasons some drugs work better than others depending on the clinical situation:

CLINICAL SITUATION	DRUG OF CHOICE
motion sickness	• scopolamine, • diphenhydramine
vertigo	• meclizine
chemotherapy	• metoclopramide
radiation therapy	• domperidone

3.55.) LAXATIVES

bulk forming [1] (stool softeners)	• fibers (fruit, vegetable) • methyl cellulose • psyllium seeds
irritants (increased intestinal motility)	• senna • castor oil
nonabsorbable salines [1] (increased osmotic pressure)	• magnesium salts
lubricants (to protect hemorrhoids)	• mineral oil

[1] *take with plenty of water*

Abuse of laxatives → *intestinal potassium loss* → *hypokalemia* →
decreased intestinal motility → *increased "need" for laxatives*

BIOCHEMISTRY

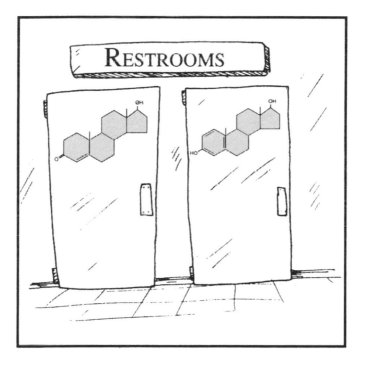

4.1.) <u>REACTIONS & LOCATIONS</u>

A) Intracellular location of some key biochemical reactions:

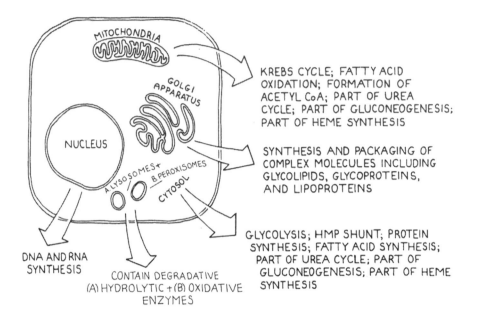

KREBS CYCLE; FATTY ACID OXIDATION; FORMATION OF ACETYL CoA; PART OF UREA CYCLE; PART OF GLUCONEOGENESIS; PART OF HEME SYNTHESIS

SYNTHESIS AND PACKAGING OF COMPLEX MOLECULES INCLUDING GLYCOLIPIDS, GLYCOPROTEINS, AND LIPOPROTEINS

GLYCOLYSIS; HMP SHUNT; PROTEIN SYNTHESIS; FATTY ACID SYNTHESIS; PART OF UREA CYCLE; PART OF GLUCONEOGENESIS; PART OF HEME SYNTHESIS

DNA AND RNA SYNTHESIS

CONTAIN DEGRADATIVE (A) HYDROLYTIC + (B) OXIDATIVE ENZYMES

B) Organ location of some key biochemical reactions:

fatty acid synthesis	liver, fat cells
gluconeogensis	liver, kidneys
heme synthesis	bone marrow
amino acid synthesis	liver
urea synthesis	liver
cholesterol synthesis	liver

Modified from Goldberg: *Clinical Biochemistry Made Ridiculously Simple*, MedMaster, 2007

4.2.) <u>ENZYME KINETICS</u>

The Lineweaver-Burke plot is a convenient way to show the relationship between **substrate concentration [S]** and **rate of reaction V**:

<u>COMPETITIVE INHIBITOR</u>: (binds at same site as substrate)

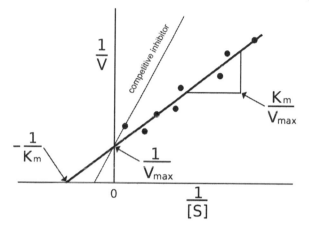

NONCOMPETITIVE INHIBITOR: (binds at different site from substrate)

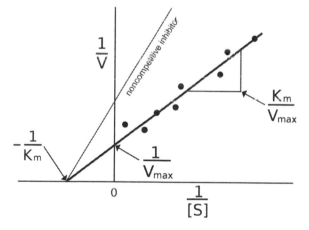

V_{max}: *Maximal rate of reaction when enzyme is saturated with substrate.*

K_m: *Substrate concentration at which reaction rate is half of its maximal value.*
High K_m = low affinity
Low K_m = high affinity

4.3.) <u>AMINO ACIDS</u>

Only 20 amino acids are commonly found in mammalian cells. Amino acids have an amino and a carboxyl group, forming peptide bonds with each other:

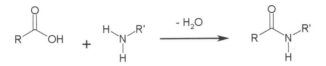

acidic	aspartate, glutamate
basic	histidine, lysine, arginine
essential	valine, leucin, isoleucine tryptophan, phenylalanine, methionine lysine, arginine histidine, threonine
strictly ketogenic	leucine, lysine
keto- and glucogenic	isoleucine, threonine tryptophan, phenylalanine

> **Glucogenic:** if carbon skeleton can be converted to glucose.
> **Ketogenic:** if carbon skeleton can be converted to acetyl CoA.

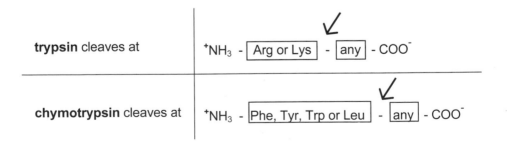

trypsin cleaves at	$^+NH_3$ - Arg or Lys - any - COO$^-$
chymotrypsin cleaves at	$^+NH_3$ - Phe, Tyr, Trp or Leu - any - COO$^-$

4.4.) <u>AMINO ACID PRECURSORS</u>

Amino acids are not only the building blocks of proteins, they are also used to form a number of biologically active molecules:

	PRODUCTS:
tyrosine	• dopa, dopamine • norepinephrine, epinephrine • T3, T4 (thyroxin) • melanin
tryptophan	• 5-HT (serotonin) • melatonin • niacin
glutamate	• GABA
glycine	• porphyrin, heme • creatine (glycine plus + arginine)
histidine	• histamine

4.5.) AMINO ACID DISORDERS

Inborn errors of metabolism prevent proper catabolism of amino acids. Most clinical symptoms are due to accumulation of metabolites.

A) ENZYMES:

	DEFECT	SIGNS & SYMPTOMS
albinism	tyrosinase	• unpigmented skin, eyes
phenylketonuria	phenylalanine hydroxylase	• mental retardation • hypopigmentation • musty odor
alkaptonuria	homogentisate oxidase	• arthritis (ochronosis) • urine darkens
maple syrup	branched chain decarboxylase	• hyperreflexia • sweet odor urine
homocystinuria	cystathionine synthetase	• mental retardation • lens dislocation

B) TRANSPORTERS: (kidneys and intestinal epithelium)

	DEFECT	SIGNS & SYMPTOMS
cystinuria	dibasic amino acid transporter	• urinary cystine stones
Hartnup disease	neutral amino acid transporter	tryptophan deficiency ↓ niacin deficiency ↓ pellagra

> **PELLAGRA** (Hartnup disease or dietary niacin deficiency):
> "3 Ds": Dermatitis, Dementia and Diarrhea

4.6.) ENZYME DEFECTS

ALBINISM: defective tyrosinase in melanocytes

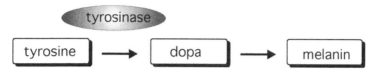

Tyrosine hydroxylase is intact...!
(Patient's nerve cells can still make dopa, epi- and norepinephrine).

PHENYLKETONURIA: defective phenylalanine hydroxylase

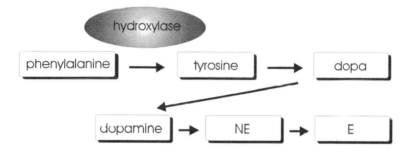

Tyrosine becomes an essential amino acid in patients with phenylketonuria.

ALKAPTONURIA: defective homogentisate oxidase

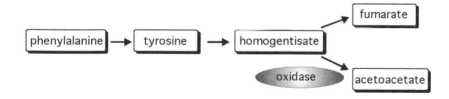

MAPLE SYRUP DISEASE: defective branched chain decarboxylase

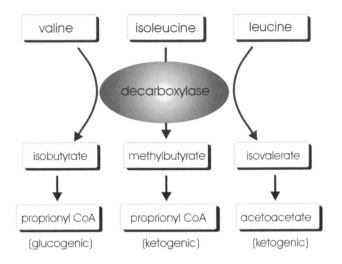

Accumulation of branched chain keto acids gives urine a sweet odor.

HOMOCYSTINURIA: defective cystathione synthase

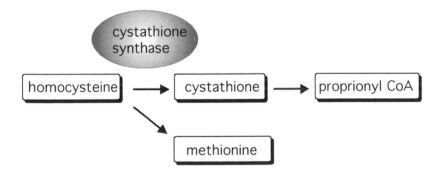

homocysteine + homocysteine → homocystine (in urine)

4.7.) <u>MONOSACCHARIDES</u>

Monosaccharides are simple sugars that are classified by the number of C atoms: pentose=5, hexose=6. There are several isomers of each sugar (i.e. same chemical formula, different configuration):

<u>EPIMERS OF GLUCOSE</u>

αD-glucose	mannose	galactose
β CHO α	CHO	CHO
2-OH	OH - 2	2-OH
OH - 3	OH - 3	OH - 3
4-OH	4-OH	OH - 4
L 5-OH D	5-OH	5-OH
CH_2OH	CH_2OH	CH_2OH

pyranose	• ring with <u>5 carbons + 1 oxygen</u> *(example: glucose)*
furanose	• ring with <u>4 carbons + 1 oxygen</u> *(example: fructose)*
anomeric carbon	• C atom that has <u>4 different ligands</u> *(for sugars this refers to the C1 in ring form)*
epimers	• **isomers that differ in only <u>one</u> carbon** *(example: glucose and galactose)*
enantiomers	• mirror image (i.e. flipped at all anomeric C atoms)
reducing sugars	• oxygen on C1 atom is available for redox reaction • glucose, galactose and fructose are reducing sugars • sucrose is a non-reducing sugar

4.8.) HEXOSE KINASES

These enzymes phosphorylate glucose to glucose-6-phosphate, which cannot get out of the cell. Glucokinase of the liver has a lower affinity, removing glucose when blood concentrations are high.

	HEXOKINASE	GLUCOKINASE
organs	muscles	liver
substrate specificity	many hexoses	many hexoses
affinity	**high**	low
V_{max} ("capacity")	low	**high**
inhibited by glucose-6 phosphate	yes	no

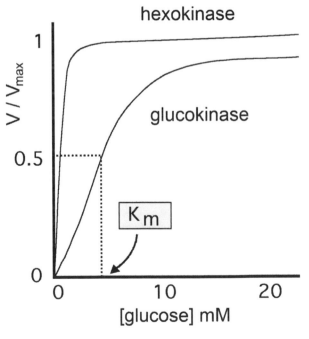

4.9.) <u>SACCHARIDES</u>

Saccharides are carbohydrates composed of several monosaccharides.

α-bond:	carbon 1 is in α position (down)
β-bond:	carbon 1 is in β position (up)

A) <u>DISACCHARIDES</u>

	COMPOSITION	BOND
maltose (beer)	glucose + glucose	α1 - 4
lactose (milk)	galactose + glucose	β1 - 4
sucrose (table sugar)	glucose + fructose	α1 - β2

B) <u>POLYSACCHARIDES</u>

	COMPOSITION	BOND
glycogen, starch	many glucoses	α1 - 4 (chains) α1 - 6 (branch points)
cellulose	many glucoses	β1 - 4

 The β1-4 bond cannot be hydrolyzed by humans. (Cellulose is indigestible).

4.10.) SACCHARIDE DISORDERS

Inborn errors of metabolism that prevent digestion or catabolism of saccharides. Clinical symptoms are mostly due to accumulation of metabolites.

	ENZYME DEFECT	SIGNS & SYMPTOMS
fructosuria	fructokinase	• benign • asymptomatic
fructose intolerance	aldolase B	• hypoglycemia • liver failure
galactosemia	uridyltransferase	• cataracts • mental retardation
lactose intolerance	lactase (usually acquired)	• diarrhea

 Diarrhea of any cause can result in temporary lactase deficiency. (Don't drink milk if you have diarrhea!)

4.11.) <u>ENZYME DEFECTS</u>

<u>FRUCTOSE INTOLERANCE</u>: defective fructokinase or aldolase-B

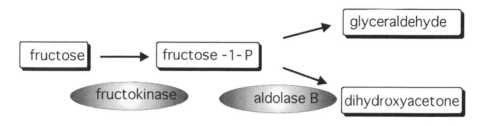

Fructosuria (defective fructokinase): Fructose is harmless.

Fructose intolerance (defective aldolase): Fructose-1-P accumulates in liver and inhibits glycogenolysis and gluconeogenesis → severe hypoglycemia.

<u>GALACTOSEMIA</u>: defective uridyltransferase

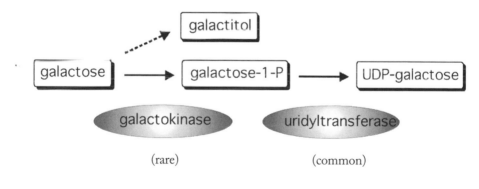

Newborn screening for this disease is mandatory, because failure to treat results in early mental retardation.

4.12.) GLYCOGEN STORAGE DISEASES

Glucose-6-phosphate cannot cross cell membranes. In Von Gierke disease, glucose-6-phosphate remains trapped inside the liver cells and inhibits glycogen breakdown.

Some glycogen is continuously degraded by lysosomal α-glucosidase. Deficiency results in glycogen accumulation in all organs.

Glycogen phosphorylase cleaves the α1-4 bond and releases glucose-1-phosphate.

	ENZYME DEFECT	ORGANS AFFECTED
Type I Von Gierke	glucose-6-phosphatase	• liver and kidneys enlarged • fasting hypoglycemia • acidosis • failure to thrive
Type II Pompe	α-glucosidase (lysosomes)	• affects all organs • muscle hypotonia • cardiac failure • death before age 2
Type V McArdle	skeletal muscle glycogen phosphorylase	• exercise: muscle pain/cramps • progressive muscle weakness

Skeletal muscle cells don't have glucose-6-phosphatase (unlike the liver, muscle cells do not release glucose into the circulation).

4.13.) <u>ENZYME DEFECTS</u>

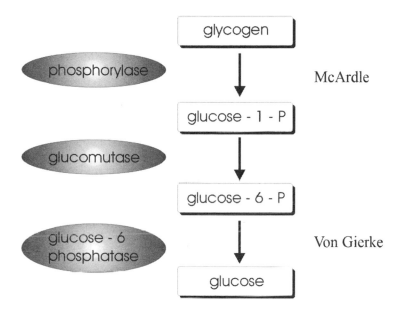

 The enzyme defect in Type II (Pompe) involves a lysosomal enzyme of an alternate pathway of glycogen breakdown.

4.14.) <u>GLYCOSAMINOGLYCANS</u>
(Mucopolysaccharides)

Long, unbranched polysaccharides composed of repeating disaccharides.
One of the disaccharides is a hexosamine (often N-acetyl-glucosamine).
They can bind large amounts of water ($\rightarrow$ gel) and provide lubrication.

GLYCOSAMINOGLYCANS
- hyaluronic acid
- heparin
- keratan sulfate
- chondroitin sulfate
- dermatan sulfate

IMPORTANT MUCOPOLYSACCHARIDOSES

	ENZYME DEFECT	SIGNS & SYMPTOMS
Hurler	α-L Iduronidase [1]	• **cornea clouding** • **mental retardation**
Scheie	α-L Iduronidase [1]	• **cornea clouding** • normal intelligence
Hunter	Iduronate sulfatase	• no clouding • **mental retardation**

[1] *same enzyme, different mutations*

PROTEOGLYCANS
- Proteoglycans have a protein core to which numerous side chains of glycosaminoglycans attach.
- Major functions: Lubricants, extracellular matrix, molecular "sieve".

4.15.) FATTY ACIDS

Fatty acids are rich in energy and needed for many physiological processes. Linoleic and arachidonic acid are "essential", i.e. cannot be synthesized by human cells. Infants should NOT be fed skim-milk formulas!

SATURATED

	STRUCTURE	FEATURES
palmitic acid	16:0	• product of human fatty acid synthesis
stearic acid	18.0	

MONOUNSATURATED (have one C=C double bond)

palmitoleic acid	16:1(9)	
oleic acid	18:1(9)	

POLYUNSATURATED (have many C=C double bonds)

linoleic acid **linolenic acid**	18:2(9,12) 18:3(9,12,15)	• plant oils
arachidonic acid	20:4(5,8,11,14)	• precursor of prostaglandins

Example: 18:1(9): 18 carbons, 1 double bond at position 9

- o Peripheral atherosclerosis correlates with saturated fat intake.
- o Margarine (hydrogenated vegetable oils = trans fatty acids) is similarly harmful.

4.16.) <u>BILE ACIDS</u>

Bile acids are amphipathic (have both polar and unpolar parts) allowing them to emulsify otherwise insoluble lipids. If bile contains more cholesterol than what can be solubilized by bile acids and phospholipids, it will crystallize and form stones.

	BILE ACIDS	FEATURES
primary	• cholic acid • chenodeoxycholic acid	• derived from cholesterol
secondary	• deoxycholic acid • lithocholic acid	• produced from primary conjugated bile salts by intestinal bacteria • less soluble → excreted
conjugate	• glycocholic acid (cholic acid + glycine) • taurocholic acid (cholic acid + taurine)	• ionized at physiologic pH • forms micelles with dietary fats

>95% of bile salts are reabsorbed in the ileum.
("Enterohepatic circulation")

4.17.) <u>LIPOPROTEINS</u>

A) Separation of lipid fractions by centrifugation and electrophoresis:

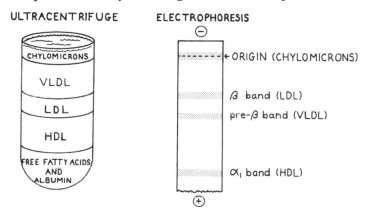

B) Distribution and fate of lipoproteins in the body:

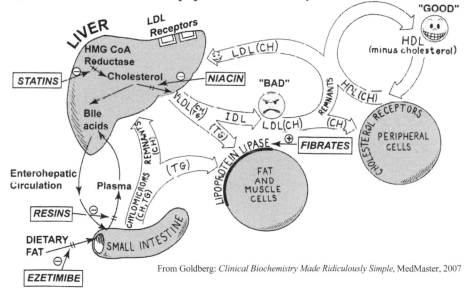

From Goldberg: *Clinical Biochemistry Made Ridiculously Simple*, MedMaster, 2007

 LDL is "bad cholesterol": increased levels increase risk for ischemic heart disease. HDL is "good cholesterol": increased levels are cardioprotective, even if LDL is low!

4.18.) PHOSPHOLIPIDS

TRIGLYCERIDES

GLYCERO-PHOSPHOLIPIDS

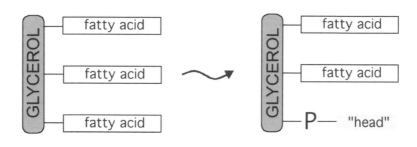

CERAMIDE

SPHINGO-PHOSPHOLIPIDS

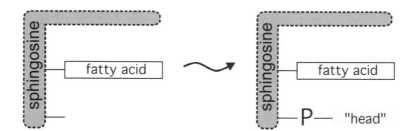

CEREBROSIDES

GANGLIOSIDES

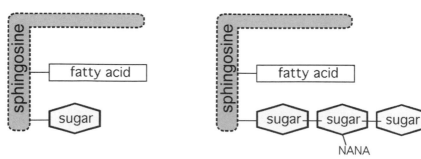

A) GLYCERO-PHOSPHOLIPIDS:
(spontaneously form lipid bilayers → cell membranes)

phosphatidyl choline (= lecithin)	phosphatidic acid + choline
phosphatidyl ethanolamine	phosphatidic acid + ethanolamine
phosphatidyl serine	phosphatidic acid + serine
phosphatidyl inositol	phosphatidic acid + inositol
cardiolipin	2x phosphatidic acid + glycerine

= "head"

B) SPHINGO-PHOSPHOLIPIDS:

ceramide	sphingosine + fatty acid
sphingomyelin	ceramide + choline

4.19.) GLYCOLIPIDS

cerebroside	ceramide + mono saccharide
globoside	ceramide + oligosaccharide
ganglioside	ceramide + oligosaccharide + NANA

4.20.) SPHINGOLIPIDOSES

Inborn errors of metabolism that prevent catabolism of sphingolipids. Clinical symptoms are due to accumulation of metabolites.

		ACCUMULATE / ENZYME	SIGNS & SYMPTOMS
Niemann-Pick	A	sphingomyelin / sphingomyelinase	• liver and spleen enlargement • foamy cells
Gaucher	A	glucocerebrosides / β-glucosidase	• liver and spleen enlargement • osteoporosis • Ashkenazi Jews
Krabbe	A	galactocerebrosides / β-galactosidase	• blindness, deafness • convulsions • globoid cells
metachromatic leukodystrophy	A	sulfatides / arylsulfatase	• progressive paralysis
Fabry	X	globosides / α-galactosidase	• reddish-purple skin rash • kidney & heart failure • angiokeratoma
Tay-Sachs	A	gangliosides / hexosaminidase	• blindness • cherry red macula • Ashkenazi Jews

A = Autosomal recessive
X = X-linked recessive

4.21.) ENZYME DEFECTS

<u>GALACTOSE</u>: defective arylsulfatase or β-galactosidase

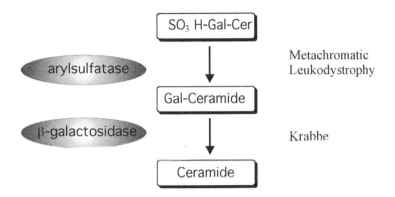

Metachromatic
Leukodystrophy

Krabbe

<u>GLUCOSE</u>: defective β-glucosidase

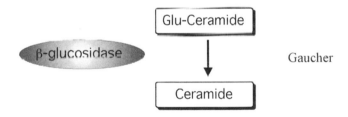

Gaucher

4.22.) <u>PORPHYRIAS</u>

Heme is an iron-containing derivative of porphyrin. Porphyrias are due to defects in heme biosynthesis and as a result precursors of heme accumulate.

	ACCUMULATE	PHOTO-SENSITIVITY	OTHER SIGNS
acute intermittent	porphobilinogen [1]	no	• **abdominal pain**
cutanea tarda	uroporphyrinogen	yes	
coproporphyria	coproporphyrinogen	yes	• **abdominal pain**
lead poisoning	δ-ALA protoporphyrin	no	• **anemia** *microcytic, hypochrome basophil stippling*

[1] *precipitated by dieting, steroids, sulfonamides and many other drugs.*

<u>MECHANISM OF PHOTOSENSITIVITY</u>:

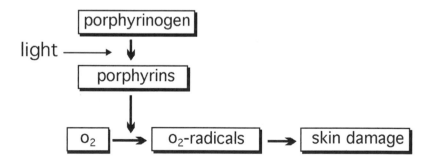

4.23.) ENYME DEFECTS

Heme is used in hemoglobin, myoglobin and cytochromes and synthesized from δ-aminolevulinic acid (glycine + succinyl CoA):

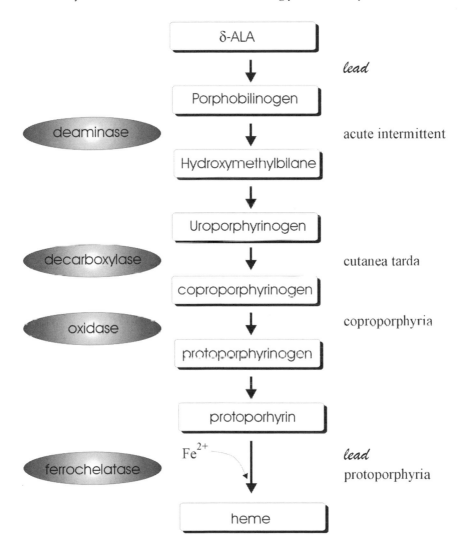

4.24.) PREFERRED NUTRIENTS

The heart is completely aerobic. In contrast, skeletal muscles can function anaerobically for some time. After a prolonged fast, metabolism adapts to preserve amino acids:

	NORMAL	PROLONGED FAST
brain	• glucose	• ketone bodies • glucose
muscle	• **rest:** fatty acids • **exercise:** glucose	• fatty acids
heart ("takes anything")	• fatty acids • ketone bodies • lactate • glucose	• fatty acids • ketone bodies • lactate • glucose
erythrocytes	• glucose	• glucose

The heart is completely aerobic. In contrast, skeletal muscles can function anaerobically for some time.

FASTING:

o The brain and red blood cells always need glucose.
o The liver maintains glucose levels by a) glycogenolysis
                                        b) gluconeogenesis

o **Substrates for liver gluconeogenesis:** Muscle, RBCs: → lactate
                                            Fat cells: triglycerides → glycerol

o **Production of ketones by liver:** Triglycerides → fatty acids → ketones

---

4.25.) <u>VITAMINS</u>

Vitamins are essential nutrients that cannot be synthesized by human cells. Deficiencies are most common in poverty and chronic alcohol abuse.

	FUNCTION	SIGNS OF DEFICIENCY
A	part of rhodopsin	night blindness (retinal) growth retardation (retinoic acid)
D	GI tract: Ca^{2+} absorption bone: supports PTH	rickets, osteomalacia
E	antioxidant	ataxia
K	carboxylation of glutamate	bleeding disorder (II, VII, IX, X)
C	hydroxylation of proline and lysine	scurvy
B1 (thiamin)	decarboxylations	beriberi
B2 (riboflavin)	flavins (FMN etc.)	glossitis, cheilosis
B6 (pyridoxine)	transaminations deaminations	anemia (microcytic) neuropathy
B12	methionine synthesis odd carbon fatty acid degradation	anemia (macrocytic) neuropathy *D. Latum* (worm infestation)
niacin	NAD^+, $NADP^+$	pellagra (=diarrhea, dementia, dermatitis)
pantothenate	Coenzyme A	headache, nausea
biotin	carboxylations	seborrheic dermatitis nervous disorders avidin (raw egg white) binds biotin
folic acid	one carbon metabolism	anemia (macrocytic) glossitis, colitis

4.26.) ATP EQUIVALENTS

Fat (9 kcal/g) is more rich in energy than protein (4 kcal/g) or sugar (4 kcal/g). Here is why:

	YIELD	EXPLANATION
FADH$_2$	2	
NADH	3	
acetyl CoA	12	acetyl CoA → 2 CO$_2$ 3 NADH + FADH$_2$ + GTP
pyruvate	15	pyruvate → acetyl CoA + NADH
glycolysis (anaerobe)	2	glucose → lactate 4 ATP minus 2 ATP [1]
glycolysis (aerobe)	8	glucose → pyruvate (4 ATP minus 2 ATP) + 2 NADH
glucose (complete oxidation)	38	glucose → 6 CO$_2$ 8 + 2x15 (pyruvate)
fatty acid (e.g. 16:0)	129	
gluconeogenesis (from pyruvate)	-12	
urea synthesis	-4	

[1] *2 ATP required for hexokinase and fructokinase reactions*

Glycerophosphate shuttle (yields 2 ATP per NADH)
Reducing equivalents are transferred from cytosolic NADH to mitochondrial FADH$_2$.

Malate shuttle (yields 3 ATP per NADH)
Reducing equivalents are transferred from cytosolic NADH to mitochondrial NADH.

4.27.) KEY ENZYMES - SUGARS

Most metabolic pathways are regulated by one or two "key enzymes" which can be allosterically activated or inhibited. Sometimes enzyme activity is dependent on phosphorylation.

CARBOHYDRATE METABOLISM:

	KEY ENZYME	ALLOSTERIC INHIBITORS	ALLOSTERIC ACTIVATORS	EFFECT OF PHOSPHORYLATION
glycolysis	phosphofructokinase-1	ATP citrate	AMP fructose 2,6 -dp	
	phosphofructokinase-2			**inhibits**
gluconeogenesis	fructosediphosphatase-1	AMP fructose 2,6 -dp	ATP citrate	
	fructosediphosphatase-2			**activates**
glycogenolysis	glycogenphosphorylase			**activates**
glycogen synthesis	glycogen synthetase			**inhibits**
pentose phosphate shunt	glucose-6-phosphate dehydrogenase	NADPH		

4.28.) KEY ENZYMES - FATS

FAT METABOLISM:

	KEY ENZYME	ALLOSTERIC INHIBITORS	ALLOSTERIC ACTIVATORS	EFFECT OF PHOSPHORYLATION
lipolysis	carnitine acyltransferase	malonyl CoA		
fat mobilization	hormone sensitive lipase			activates
lipid synthesis	acetyl-CoA carboxylase		citrate	inhibits
cholesterol synthesis	HMG CoA reductase		cholesterol	inhibits

4.29.) KEY ENZYMES - OTHERS

OTHER PATHWAYS:

	KEY ENZYME	ALLOSTERIC INHIBITORS	EFFECT OF PHOSPHORYLATION
ketone body synthesis	HMG CoA synthase		
purine synthesis	amidotransferase	AMP GMP IMP	
citric acid cycle	pyruvate dehydrogenase 1	Acetyl CoA NADH	**inhibits**
	citrate synthase [2]	Acetyl CoA ATP NADH	

4.30.) STEROIDS

Steroid hormones are made from cholesterol:

CLASS	EXAMPLE	NUMBER OF C-ATOMS
sterols	cholesterol	27
bile acids	glycocholate taurocholate	24
glucocorticoids	cortisol	21
mineralocorticoids	aldosterone	21
gestagens	progesterone	21
androgens	testosterone * androstenedione DHEAS	19
estrogens	estradiol * estriol	18

most potent

17-ketosteroids (dehydroandrosterone and androstenedione) ↑
- 11-hydroxylase deficiency
- 21-hydroxylase deficiency
- Cushing's syndrome
- androgen producing adrenal or gonadal tumors

17-hydroxysteroids (cortisol metabolites) ↑
- 11-hydroxylase deficiency
- Cushing's syndrome

4.31.) <u>ADRENAL GLAND</u>

Steroid synthesis always follows the same scheme, but different tissues have different sets of enzymes, resulting in different products:

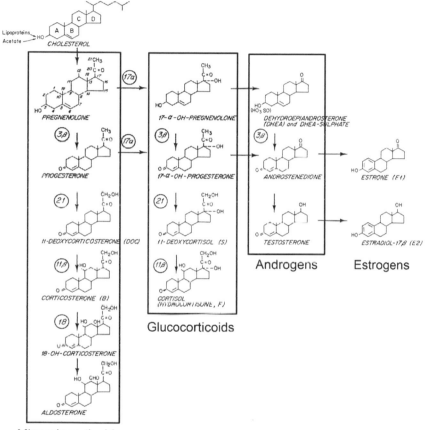

Mineralocorticoids   Glucocorticoids   Androgens   Estrogens

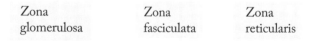

4.32.) <u>TESTIS (Leydig Cells)</u>

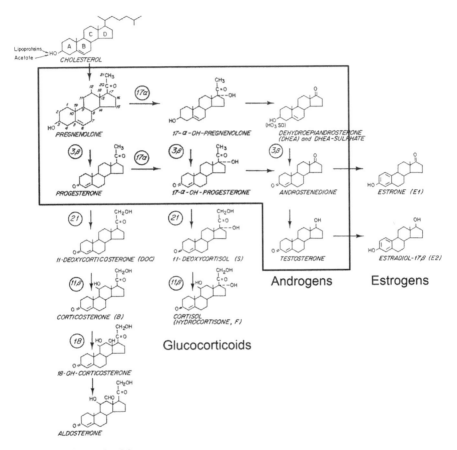

CHOLESTEROL

Lipoproteins
Acetate

PREGNENOLONE

17-α-OH-PREGNENOLONE

DEHYDROEPIANDROSTERONE
(DHEA) and DHEA-SULPHATE

PROGESTERONE

17-α-OH-PROGESTERONE

ANDROSTENEDIONE

ESTRONE (E1)

11-DEOXYCORTICOSTERONE (DOC)

11-DEOXYCORTISOL (S)

TESTOSTERONE

ESTRADIOL-17β (E2)

CORTICOSTERONE (B)

CORTISOL
(HYDROCORTISONE, F)

Androgens

Estrogens

18-OH-CORTICOSTERONE

Glucocorticoids

ALDOSTERONE

Mineralocorticoids

4.33.) <u>PERIPHERAL METABOLISM</u>

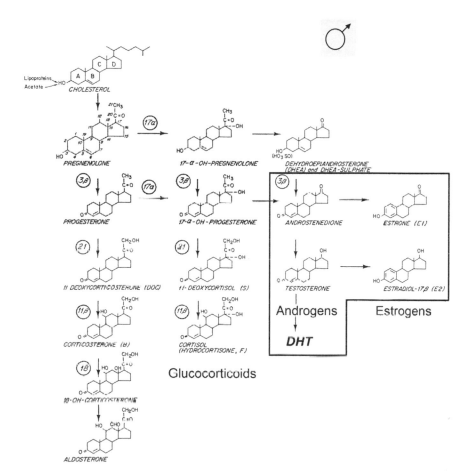

CHOLESTEROL

PREGNENOLONE

17-α-OH-PREGNENOLONE

DEHYDROEPIANDROSTERONE
(DHEA) and DHEA-SULPHATE

PROGESTERONE

17-α-OH-PROGESTERONE

ANDROSTENEDIONE

ESTRONE (E1)

11 DEOXYCORTICOSTERONE (DOC)

11-DEOXYCORTISOL (S)

TESTOSTERONE

ESTRADIOL-17β (E2)

CORTICOSTERONE (B)

CORTISOL
(HYDROCORTISONE, F)

Androgens

Estrogens

DHT

Glucocorticoids

18-OH-CORTICOSTERONE

ALDOSTERONE

Mineralocorticoids

239

4.34.) <u>OVARY (Theca Cells)</u>

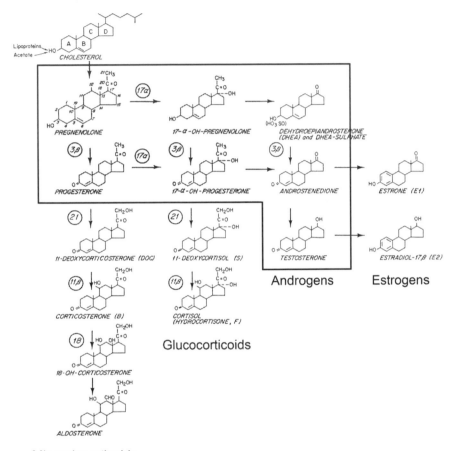

Androgens   Estrogens

Glucocorticoids

Mineralocorticoids

4.35.) <u>OVARY (Granulosa Cells)</u>

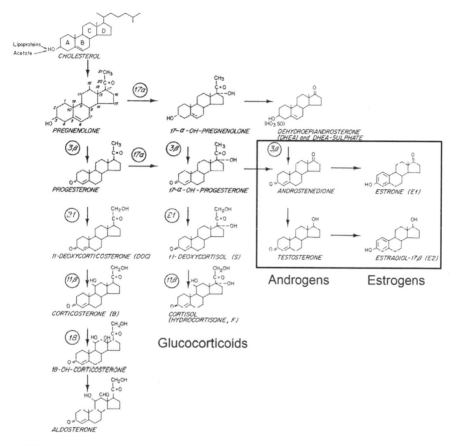

Androgens   Estrogens

Glucocorticoids

Mineralocorticoids

241

4.36.) <u>PERIPHERAL METABOLISM</u>

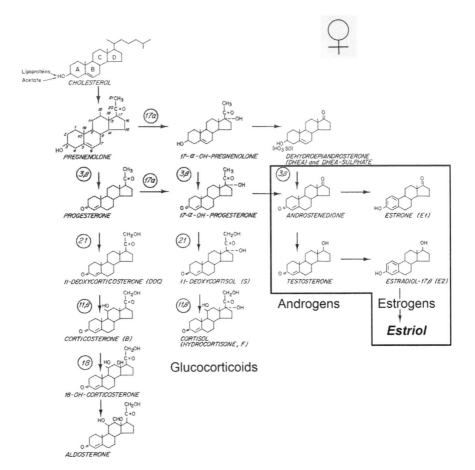

CHOLESTEROL

PREGNENOLONE — 17-α-OH-PREGNENOLONE — DEHYDROEPIANDROSTERONE (DHEA) and DHEA-SULPHATE

PROGESTERONE — 17-α-OH-PROGESTERONE — ANDROSTENEDIONE — ESTRONE (E1)

11-DEOXYCORTICOSTERONE (DOC) — 11-DEOXYCORTISOL (S) — TESTOSTERONE — ESTRADIOL-17,β (E2)

CORTICOSTERONE (B) — CORTISOL (HYDROCORTISONE, F)

18-OH-CORTICOSTERONE

ALDOSTERONE

Androgens   Estrogens
                       ↓
                   Estriol

Glucocorticoids

Mineralocorticoids

242

4.37.) <u>CORPUS LUTEUM</u>

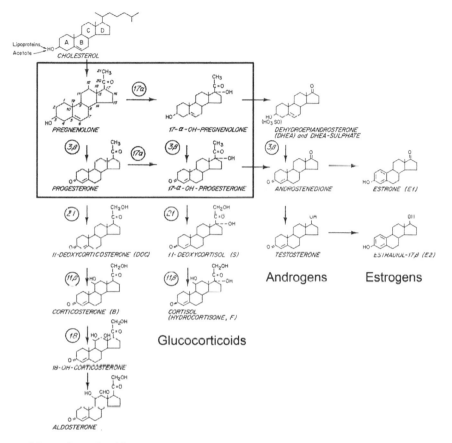

Androgens   Estrogens

Glucocorticoids

Mineralocorticoids

4.38.) 17-α-HYDROXYLASE DEFICIENCY

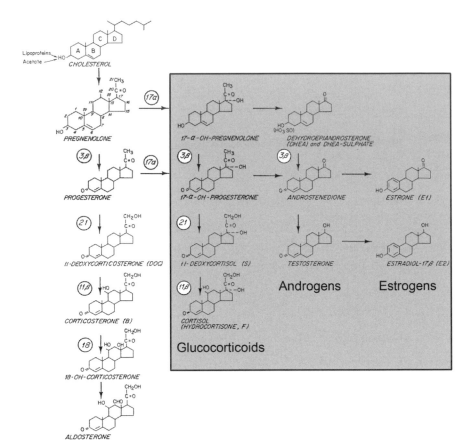

Mineralocorticoids

Male:	ambiguous genitalia
Female:	primary amenorrhea at puberty

4.39.) 21-α-HYDROXYLASE DEFICIENCY

most common defect of
corticoid synthesis (95%)

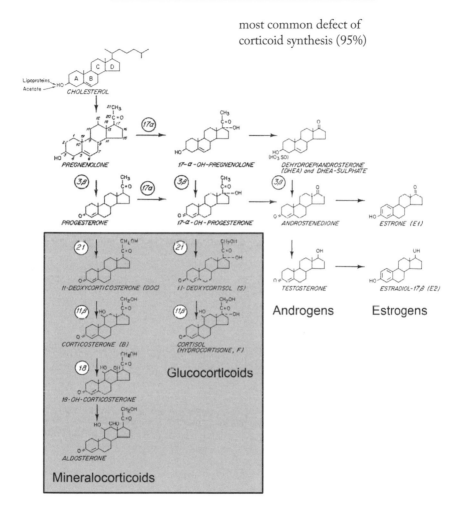

Male:	precocious puberty (DHEA↑)
Female:	ambiguous genitalia (DHEA↑)
Salt wasting:	50-60% of patients (lack of aldosterone)

4.40.) 11-β-HYDROXYLASE

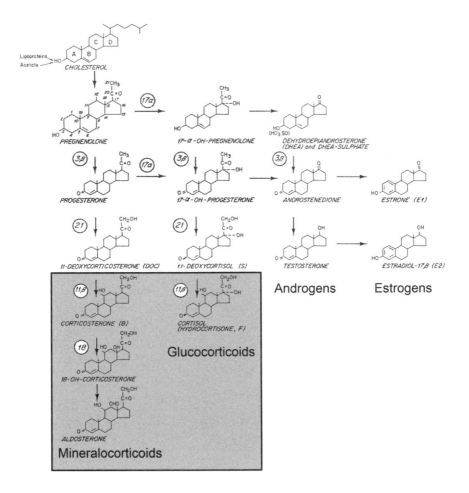

Male:	precocious puberty (androgens↑)
Female:	ambiguous genitalia (androgens↑)
Salt retention:	hypertension, hypokalemia
	(deoxycorticosterone has mineralocorticoid action)

4.41.) ENDOCRINE CONTROL OF METABOLISM

	fat	sugar	proteins
insulin	(A) • synthesis	(A) • uptake (M,F) • glycolysis (L,M) • glycogen synthesis (L,M)	(A) • synthesis
glucagon	(C) • lysis	(C) • gluconeogenesis (L) • glycogenolysis (L)	(C) • increases uptake of AA in liver for gluconeogenesis
GH	(C) • lysis	(C) • gluconeogenesis (L)	(A) • synthesis
cortisol	(C) • lysis • redistribution	(A) • inhibits uptake (M,F) • gluconeogenesis (L) • glycogen synthesis (L)	(C) • degradation
epinephrine	(C) • lysis	(C) • increases uptake (M) • glycolysis (M) • gluconeogenesis (L) • glycogenolysis (L,M)	-

(A) = anabolic   (C) = catabolic   M = Muscle   L = Liver   F = Fat

➤ **Insulin** has a general anabolic action
➤ **GH** promotes synthesis of protein at the expense fat and sugars.
➤ **Cortisol** increases blood sugar levels and build-up of glycogen stores at the expense of fat and protein

4.42.) <u>NUCLEOTIDES</u>

Nucleosides are purines or pyrimidines linked to a pentose sugar.
Nucleotides are phosphates (mono-, di- or tri-) of the nucleoside.

BASE	NUCLEOSIDE	NUCLEOTIDE
PURINES		
• adenine	• adenosine	• adenylate (AMP)
• guanine	• guanosine	• guanylate (GMP)
PYRIMIDINES		
• uracil	• uridine	• uridylate (UMP)
• cytosine	• cytidine	• cytidylate (CMP)
• thymine	• deoxythymidine	• deoxythymidylate (dTMP)

Thymidine   AZT

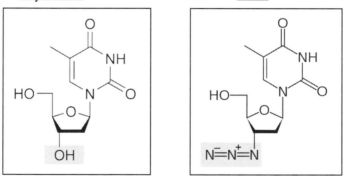

*AZT (Zidovudine) can be incorporated into the HIV DNA transcript by
viral reverse transcriptase.
Lack of the 3'-OH group then inhibits further elongation of HIV DNA.*

Mammalian polymerase is less likely to mistake AZT for thymidine.

4.43.) PURINES

Purines can either be made from scratch ("de novo") from amino acids, or they can be recycled. Recycling is especially important for tissues with rapid cell turnover (blood cells, epithelia…)

A) De novo synthesis (in liver):

1.) | phosphoribosyl pyrophosphate | → | IMP |

2.) | IMP | → | AMP or GMP | → | ADP or GDP |

B) Salvage of purine bases (recycling):

| hypoxanthine | → | IMP |

| guanine | → | GMP |

| adenine | → | AMP |

 Lesch-Nyhan: *Defective phosphoribosyl transferase: Purine bases cannot be salvaged and are all degraded to uric acid → gout, severe neurological signs.*

C) Degradation of purine bases (in liver):

1.) | adenosine | → | inosine | → | hypoxanthine | → | xanthine |

| guanosine | → | guanine | → | xanthine |

2.) | xanthine | → | uric acid |

 Allopurinol *inhibits conversion of xanthine to uric acid and is used for treatment of gout.*

4.44.) PYRIMIDINES

Like the purines, pyrimidines can be made "from scratch" or recycled:

A) De novo synthesis (in liver):

1.) $\boxed{\text{glutamine}} \rightarrow \boxed{\text{carbamoylphosphate}} \rightarrow \boxed{\text{OMP}} \rightarrow \boxed{\text{UMP}}$

2.) $\boxed{\text{UTP}} \rightarrow \boxed{\text{CTP}}$

$\boxed{\text{dUMP}} \rightarrow \boxed{\text{dTMP}}$

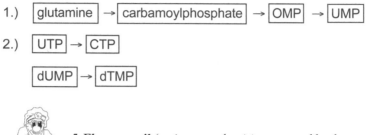

5-Fluorouracil (anti cancer drug) is converted by these same enzymes to 5-FdUMP which is a potent inhibitor of thymidine synthesis.

B) Salvage of pyrimidine bases ("recycling"):

$\boxed{\text{uracil}} \rightarrow \boxed{\text{UMP}}$

$\boxed{\text{cytosine}} \rightarrow \boxed{\text{CMP}}$

C) Degradation of pyrimidine bases (in liver):

Pyrimidine rings can be opened and completely degraded:

$\boxed{\text{cytosine}} \rightarrow CO_2, NH_4^+$ and β-alanine

$\boxed{\text{thymine}} \rightarrow CO_2, NH_4^+$ and β-amino-isobutyrate

These degradation products are harmless and are excreted in the urine.

4.45.) <u>GENE EXPRESSION</u>

When studying molecular biology, you must pay close attention to differences between prokaryotes and eukaryotes. While the principles are the same, the details are quite different.

A) <u>BACTERIA (PROKARYOTES)</u>:

operon (DNA)	• operational unit that is either "on" or "off" • consists of promoter, operator and one or more structural genes
promoter (DNA)	• RNA polymerase binds to promoter • located 5'-end of operon ("upstream")
operator (DNA)	• located between promoter and structural genes • binding site of repressors • if repressor binds to operator, the operon is "off" (polymerase can't proceed)
repressor (protein)	• regulatory protein that binds to operator and prevents transcription
regulator gene (DNA)	• codes for repressor

---

lac-OPERON:
➤ Metabolite (lactose) binds to repressor preventing its interaction with DNA.
➤ Operon freed of repressor is switched "on" and polymerase begins transcription of structural genes.
➤ Gene products: β-galactosidase plus two other proteins

B) HUMANS (EUKARYOTES):

- No operon. Each structural gene has its own promoter containing many different response elements (binding sites for regulatory proteins).

- Regulatory proteins can bind to several promoters activating a set of structural genes (which may be located on different chromosomes).

- Transcription is regulated by various combinations of regulatory proteins.

transcription factor	• binds to TATA box (part of promoter) • RNA polymerase does not recognize promoter in absence of transcription factor!
inducers	• example: steroid hormones • bind to nuclear receptor protein • inducer-receptor complex binds to DNA and activates some gene, inactivates others
enhancers	• regulatory DNA sequence • can be upstream or downstream of promoter • may be located several thousand base pairs from starting point of transcription • loops in DNA bring enhancers near the promoter region of the gene

4.46.) <u>TRANSCRIPTION</u>
DNA → RNA

mRNA are the "working copies" of the DNA. While cells from different tissues of the body have the same DNA, they differ in their gene expression and have different sets of mRNA. If you want to know which genes are active, you can make a cDNA library (complimentary DNA synthesized to all mRNA present in a cell).

A) <u>BACTERIA (PROKARYOTES)</u>:

holoenzyme	• core enzyme plus σ-factor
σ-factors	• bind to RNA polymerase. • depending on σ-factor, RNA polymerase • recognizes certain promoters but not others
cistron	• region of DNA that encodes a single protein

Prokaryotic mRNA is polycistronic (encodes multiple proteins).

B) <u>HUMANS (EUKARYOTES)</u>:

polymerase I	• makes rRNA
polymerase II	• makes mRNA
polymerase III	• makes tRNA

Eukaryotic mRNA is heavily processed in the nucleus:
1. *5'-cap (methylated GTP) is added.*
2. *Poly (A) tail is added to 3' end.*
3. *Introns are removed and exons are spliced together.*

4.47.) REPLICATION
DNA → DNA

Replication of eukaryotic DNA is <u>semiconservative</u>: parental strands separate and each serves as a template for a newly synthesized one. DNA polymerases cannot initiate synthesis of a new strand but require a <u>primer</u> (short oligonucleotide sequence composed of RNA). The primer later needs to be replaced by DNA.

> ➤ Parental strand is read in 3' to 5' direction.
> ➤ New strand is produced in 5' to 3' direction.

A) BACTERIA (PROKARYOTES):

helicase	• separates parental DNA
primase	• RNA polymerase that copies parental strand and makes RNA primer
polymerase III	• major DNA polymerase • replicates both parental strands • has proofreading ability • has 3' exonuclease activity to remove wrong nucleotides
polymerase I	• removes primer and fills gap with DNA (5' exonuclease activity)
polymerase II	• DNA repair (3' exonuclease activity)
ligase	• joins Okazaki fragments of lagging strand

B) HUMANS (EUKARYOTES):

δ	• major DNA polymerase
	• produces leading strand
	• also has helicase activity!
	  ○ *no proofreading*
	  ○ *no exonuclease activity*

α	• DNA polymerase • produces lagging strand ○ *also has primase activity!*
β, ε	• minor DNA polymerases • DNA repair (3' exonuclease activity)
γ	• mitochondrial DNA polymerase
ligase	• joins Okazaki fragments of lagging strand

> ➢ **Endonuclease:** Incision of DNA
> ➢ **Exonuclease:** Removal of nucleotides from incised end

ANATOMY

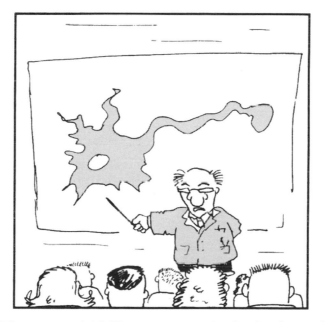

"There are 14 billion neurons in the brain and 14 billion *and one* facts to remember to pass the USMLE exams."

Part A : Embryology

5.1.) GERM LAYERS

All tissues are derived from 3 embryonal germ cell layers. Adenomas and carcinomas develop in organs derived from ecto- or endoderm, sarcomas and fibromas in organs derived from the mesoderm.

ECTODERM	• **neural tube** → CNS • **neural crest** → peripheral nervous system • **placodes** → sensory organs • **surface** epithelium → skin
MESODERM	• **somites** → muscles, vertebral column • connective tissue • lymphatic tissues • blood cells
ENDODERM	• epithelium of GI tract • liver • pancreas • thymus • thyroid

5.2.) <u>FETAL REMNANTS</u>

The umbilical cord contains 2 arteries (deoxygenated blood) and 1 vein (oxygenated blood from placenta). The yolk stalk connects the yolk sac with the GI tract, the urachus connects the urinary bladder with the allantois. These fetal structures disappear and leave remnants.

umbilical arteries	medial umbilical ligaments
urachus	median umbilical ligament
umbilical vein	round ligament
ductus venosus	venous ligament
ductus arteriosus	ligamentum arteriosus
yolk stalk	Meckel's diverticulum

<u>Meckel's diverticulum</u>: "2-2-2"
- persists in **2%** of persons
- located at antimesenteric border of ileum (within **2** feet of the ileocecal junction)
- is about **2** cm long

Inflammation may mimic appendicitis!

5.3.) DERIVATES OF BRANCHIAL ARCHES

Branchial arches form the pharynx-neck region (gills) of vertebrates. Each arch consists of a mesenchymal core covered by ectoderm (outside) and endoderm (inside) and gives rise to a specific bones, muscles, arteries and nerves:

	BONES	MUSCLES	ARTERIES	NERVES
1st Arch mandibular arch (Meckel)	malleus incus	muscles of mastication	facial artery	V3
2nd Arch hyoid arch (Reichert)	stapes styloid lesser horns of hyoid	muscles of facial expression	ext. carotid artery	VII
3rd Arch thyrohyoid arch	body of hyoid	stylopharyngeal muscle	int. carotid artery	IX
4th Arch	larynx	pharyngeal muscles		X

PHARYNGEAL CLEFTS:
I: (between arch I and II) - forms external auditory meatus
II-IV: - cervical sinus (disappears, but may form cervical cysts)

5.4.) <u>PHARYNGEAL POUCHES</u>

Each of the pharyngeal clefts separating the branchial arches has a corresponding pouch on the inside. The clefts disappear (except for I) while the pouches give off specialized tissues:

	TISSUES DERIVED FROM POUCHES
I	tympanic cavity eustachian tube
II	palatine tonsil
III	ventral: thymus dorsal: <u>inferior</u> parathyroids
IV	ventral: - dorsal: <u>superior</u> parathyroids
V	ultimobranchial body → parafollicular C cells of thyroid

<u>Cervical cysts:</u>
- *uncommon remnants of pharyngeal clefts*
- *located in anterolateral part of neck*
- *1-2 inches in diameter*

5.5.) UROGENITAL DEVELOPMENT

Up to the 7th week, the embryo is ambisexual and contains both Wolff and Müller ducts:

	MALE	FEMALE
Wolff [1]	• epididymis • vas deferens	disappears
Müller [2]	disappears	• fallopian tubes • uterus • vagina down to hymen

[1] = *mesonephric duct*
[2] = *paramesonephric duct*

MALE DIFFERENTIATION:
Wolff is sustained by testosterone (from Leydig cells)
Müller is suppressed by MIF glycoprotein (from Sertoli cells)

---

allantois	• urinary bladder • urachus
ureteric bud[1]	• bladder trigonum • ureter • collecting tubules
pronephros	(disappears, never functional)
mesonephros	(disappears, temporarily functional)
metanephros	• kidneys

[1] *inferior part of mesonephric duct (= metanephric duct)*

5.6.) <u>FETAL CIRCULATION</u>

Fetal:

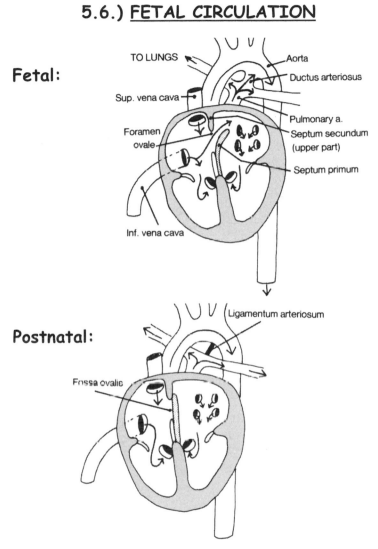

TO LUNGS
Aorta
Ductus arteriosus
Sup. vena cava
Pulmonary a.
Foramen ovale
Septum secundum (upper part)
Septum primum
Inf. vena cava

Postnatal:

Ligamentum arteriosum
Fossa ovalis

From Goldberg: *Clinical Anatomy Made Ridiculously Simple*, MedMaster, 2007

Which vessels carry oxygenated blood, which carry mixed blood, and which carry unoxygenated venous blood? Also see Physiology 6.29

Part B : Gross Anatomy

5.7.) THE SKULL AND ITS HOLES

optic canal	• optic nerve • ophthalmic artery
superior orbital fissure	• cranial nerves III, IV, V (ophthalmic), VI • sympathetic nerves • ophthalmic veins
foramen rotundum	• cranial nerve V (maxillary)
foramen ovale	• cranial nerve V (mandibular) • accessory meningeal artery
foramen spinosum	• middle meningeal artery
foramen magnum	• spinal cord • accessory nerve • vertebral arteries • spinal arteries
jugular foramen	• cranial nerves IX, X, XI • internal jugular vein
hypoglossal canal	• cranial nerve XII
internal auditory meatus	• cranial nerves VII, VIII • labyrinthine artery

 Basilar skull fractures: bruises over mastoid process or periorbital.

5.8.) EYE

The eye is moved by 6 external muscles, innervated by 3 cranial nerves:

A) EXTERNAL MUSCLES:

MUSCLE	MOVES EYE:	INNERVATION
med. rectus	nasal	III (oculomotor)
lat. rectus	temporal	VI (abducens)

combined action raises eye upward:

sup. rectus	**up and nasal** rotates medially	III
inf. oblique	**up and temporal** rotates laterally	III

combined action lowers eye downward:

inf. rectus	**down and nasal** rotates laterally	III
sup. oblique	**down and temporal** rotates medially	IV (trochlear)

__Abducens paralysis__: → *unable to abduct eye on affected side*
→ *diplopia (double vision)*

__Trochlear paralysis__: → *slight vertical double image*
→ *patient compensates by tilting head*

B) INTERNAL MUSCLES:

	FUNCTION	INNERVATION
dilator pupillae	mydriasis	sympathetic
sphincter pupillae	miosis	parasympathetic
ciliary muscle	accommodation	parasympathetic

Contraction of the ciliary muscle relaxes suspensory ligaments and allows lens to turn into globular shape for near vision.

C) UPPER EYELIDS:

	FUNCTION	INNERVATION
levator palpebrae sup.	raises lid	III (oculomotor)
Müller's muscle	raises lid	sympathetic

Drowsiness → reduced sympathetic tone
→ Müller's muscles relax
→ eyelids droop

HORNER'S SYNDROME
Caused by neck injuries or tumors interrupting cervical sympathetic chain.
1. *miosis* (small pupils)
2. *ptosis* (drooping eyelid)
3. red and dry facial skin on affected side

5.9.) TONGUE

A) MUSCLES:

The tongue is moved by three muscles, all of which are innervated by the hypoglossal nerve (XII):

MUSCLES	FUNCTION
genioglossus	pulls tongue out
styloglossus	pulls tongue in and up
hyoglossus	pulls tongue down

DAMAGE TO HYPOGLOSSAL NERVE (XII):
- genioglossus muscle of healthy side becomes dominant
- tongue will deviate <u>towards</u> side of damage

B) SENSATION:

The tongue receives sensory innervation from 3 cranial nerves:

	TASTE	TOUCH, TEMPERATURE
anterior 2/3	VII	V3
posterior 1/3	IX	IX

5.10.) <u>MANDIBLE</u>

The mandible is the largest and strongest bone in the face. In old age it atrophies somewhat as teeth are lost. The mandible and the muscles that move it are derived from the 1st branchial arch.

MUSCLES	FUNCTION
• **lat. pterygoid** • **digastric** • **geniohyoid**	open mouth
• **masseter** • medial pterygoid • temporalis	close mouth
• **lateral pterygoid**	protrudes mandible
• **temporalis**	retracts mandible
• **lateral pterygoid**	lateral displacement

 A blow to the jaw may fracture the neck of the mandible and/or the region of the opposite canine tooth.

5.11.) LARYNX

The larynx consists of 4 cartilages: The cricoid and thyroid cartilages plus a pair of arytenoid cartilages to which the vocal cords are attached. The epiglottis cartilage forms the roof and protects the larynx during swallowing.

A) MUSCLES:

	FUNCTION	INNERVATION
post. cricoarytenoid	opens glottis	recurrent nerve
lat. cricoarytenoid	closes glottis	recurrent nerve
thyroarytenoid	relaxes vocal chords	recurrent nerve
cricothyroid	tightens vocal chords	sup. laryngeal nerve

Recurrent nerves are vulnerable to injury:
- thyroidectomy
- carotid endarterectomy
- other operations in anterior triangle of the neck

unilateral damage → hoarseness
bilateral damage → dyspnea

Left recurrent nerve wraps around aortic arch
Right recurrent nerve wraps around right subclavian artery

B) SENSATION: These nerves are important to initiate the cough reflex.

above glottis	sup. laryngeal nerve
below glottis	recurrent nerve

5.12.) <u>SHOULDER</u>

Many muscles are involved in every movement. This chart lists only the <u>main</u> muscle responsible for each movement:

FUNCTION	MAIN MUSCLE	INNERVATION
adduction	pectoralis major	C5-T1
abduction	first 60 degrees: deltoid then: serratus anterior	long thoracic nerve
anteversion	deltoid	axillary nerve
retroversion	teres major	subscapular nerve
outward rotation	infraspinatus	suprascapular nerve
inward rotation	subscapular	subscapular nerve

"SCAPULA WINGING" (paralysis of anterior serratus muscle):
- damage to the long thoracic nerve (stab wounds, thoracic surgery)
- medial border of scapula stands out when the person presses his arm anteriorly against a wall.

<u>ROTATOR CUFF</u>: **supraspinatus,   infraspinatus**
teres minor,   subscapularis

- These muscles hold the head of humerus in glenoid cavity of scapula.
- Injury results in instability of the shoulder joint.

Inflammation of subacromial bursa → pain intensifies by abduction.

MUSCLES CONNECTING SCAPULA TO TRUNK:

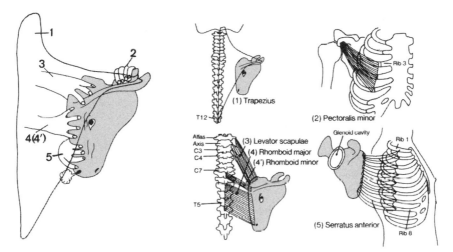

(1) Trapezius

(2) Pectoralis minor

(3) Levator scapulae
(4) Rhomboid major
(4') Rhomboid minor

(5) Serratus anterior

MUSCLES CONNECTING HUMERUS TO SCAPULA:

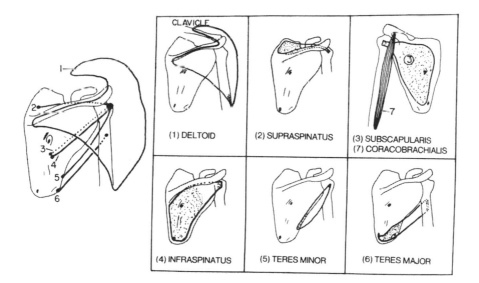

(1) DELTOID

(2) SUPRASPINATUS

(3) SUBSCAPULARIS
(7) CORACOBRACHIALIS

(4) INFRASPINATUS

(5) TERES MINOR

(6) TERES MAJOR

From Goldberg: *Clinical Anatomy Made Ridiculously Simple*, MedMaster, 2007

5.13.) BRACHIAL PLEXUS

You don't need to know every detail about the brachial plexus.
There are 3 trunks distributing to 5 major nerves:

SPINAL RAMI	TRUNKS	TERMINAL NERVES
C5 - C6	upper trunk	musculocutaneous nerve
C7	middle trunk	axillary nerve radial nerve median nerve
C8 - T1	lower trunk	ulnar nerve

⌷⌷⌷⌷ = posterior cord

5.14.) BRACHIAL PLEXUS INJURIES

These occur sometimes during delivery of a baby, if you pull the arm too much

◀

upper brachial plexus injury	• forceful separation of neck and shoulder • motorcycle accidents, football tackling • arm hangs in medial rotation **("waiter's tip position")**
posterior cord injury	• compression by too long crutches • radial nerve injury **("wrist drop")**
lower brachial plexus injury	• forceful pull of arm/shoulders (birth) • ulnar nerve injury **("claw hand")**

5.15.) BRACHIAL NERVE INJURIES

Injury to brachial nerves results in characteristic motor and sensory deficits.

	NERVE INJURY RESULTS IN:
radial nerve	• **"wrist drop"** • loss of triceps reflex ○ *sensory loss: posterior arm, dorsal hand*
median nerve	• no flexion of thumb, index and middle finger • no thumb opposition • thenar atrophy ○ *sensory loss: radial 2½ fingers (palm and tips)*
ulnar nerve	• **"claw hand"** • no flexion of 4th and 5th finger • apothenar atrophy ○ *sensory loss: ulnar 1½ fingers (palm and tips)*
musculocutaneous n.	• no elbow flexion • no supination • loss of biceps reflex ○ *sensory loss: extensor aspect of forearm*

Carpal tunnel syndrome: Compression of <u>median nerve</u> by carpal ligament.
→ pain/tingling in distribution area of median nerve (often most bothersome at night)

Humerus fracture: Risk of <u>radial nerve</u> injury (spirals down near humerus).

5.16.) <u>ELBOW</u>

This chart lists only the <u>main</u> muscle responsible for each movement:

FUNCTION	MAIN MUSCLE	INNERVATION
flexion	biceps brachii	musculocutaneous nerve
extension	triceps brachii	radial nerve
supination [1]	biceps brachii	musculocutaneous nerve
pronation [2]	pronator teres	median nerve

[1] *palm faces anteriorly, thumb points to lateral side*
[2] *palm faces posteriorly, thumb points to medial side*

"TENNIS ELBOW"
- repetitive stress, especially "backhand play"
- due to inflammation of the lateral epicondyle, which is the origin of extensor muscles of the forearm.
- elbow joint and olecranon are NOT involved!

Colles' fracture: *Fracture of radius near wrist*
→ *dorsal/lateral position of hand*

MUSCLES FLEXING THE ELBOW:

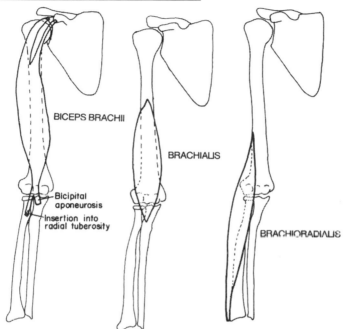

BICEPS BRACHII

BRACHIALIS

Bicipital aponeurosis

Insertion into radial tuberosity

BRACHIORADIALIS

MUSCLES FLEXING WIRST AND FINGERS:

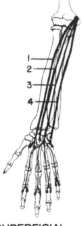

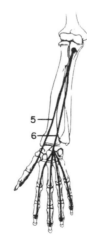

(1) FLEXOR CARPI RADIALIS (flexes, abducts wrist)
(2) PALMARIS LONGUS (flexes wrist)
(3) FLEXOR DIGITORUM SUPERFICIALIS (flexes wrist & medial 4 digits at middle phalanx)
(4) FLEXOR CARPI ULNARIS (flexes & adducts wrist)
(5) FLEXOR POLLICIS LONGUS (flexes thumb)
(6) FLEXOR DIGITORUM PROFUNDUS (flexes wrist & medial 4 digits at distal phalanx)

A. SUPERFICIAL MUSCLES

B. DEEP MUSCLES

From Goldberg: *Clinical Anatomy Made Ridiculously Simple*, MedMaster, 2007

275

MAIN NERVES OF ARM:

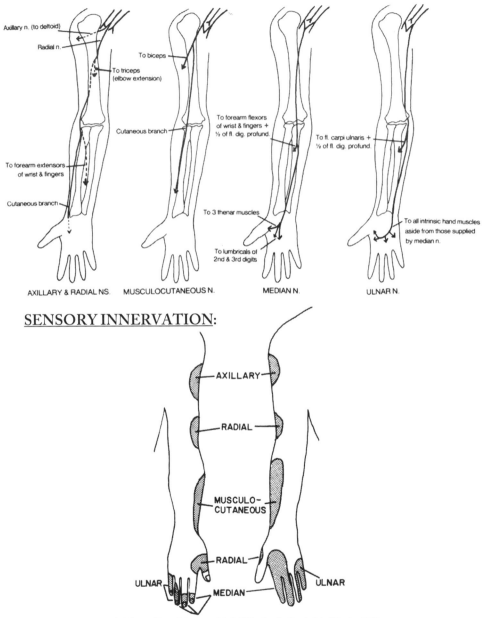

Axillary n. (to deltoid)

Radial n.

To biceps

To triceps
(elbow extension)

To forearm flexors
of wrist & fingers +
½ of fl. dig. profund.

To fl. carpi ulnaris +
½ of fl. dig. profund.

Cutaneous branch

To forearm extensors
of wrist & fingers

Cutaneous branch

To 3 thenar muscles

To all intrinsic hand muscles
aside from those supplied
by median n.

To lumbricals of
2nd & 3rd digits

AXILLARY & RADIAL NS.   MUSCULOCUTANEOUS N.   MEDIAN N.   ULNAR N.

SENSORY INNERVATION:

AXILLARY

RADIAL

MUSCULO-
CUTANEOUS

RADIAL

ULNAR

MEDIAN

ULNAR

From Goldberg: *Clinical Anatomy Made Ridiculously Simple*, MedMaster, 2007

276

5.17.) <u>WRIST CUTS</u>

Attempted suicide damages many structures in the wrist before the patient reaches the deep lying arteries…:

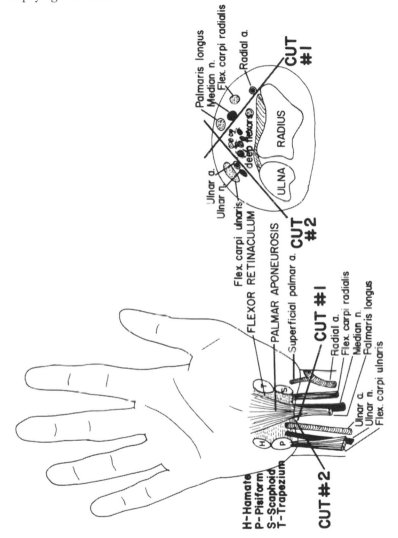

From Goldberg: *Clinical Anatomy Made Ridiculously Simple*, MedMaster, 2007

5.18.) HIP

This chart lists only the __main__ muscle responsible for each movement:

FUNCTION	MAIN MUSCLE	INNERVATION
outward rotation	gluteus maximus	inf. gluteal nerve
inward rotation	gluteus medius / minimus	sup. gluteal nerve
extension	gluteus maximus	inf. gluteal nerve
flexion	iliopsoas	femoral nerve
abduction	gluteus medius	sup. gluteal nerve
adduction	adductor magnus / minimus	obturator nerve

Pelvic fractures:	• automobile accidents • risk of severe internal bleeding
Femur neck fractures:	• common in elderly women (osteoporosis) • risk of femur head necrosis • significant morbidity / mortality

 Femur neck fracture*: the leg is abducted and externally rotated.*

MEDIAL THIGH MUSCLES:

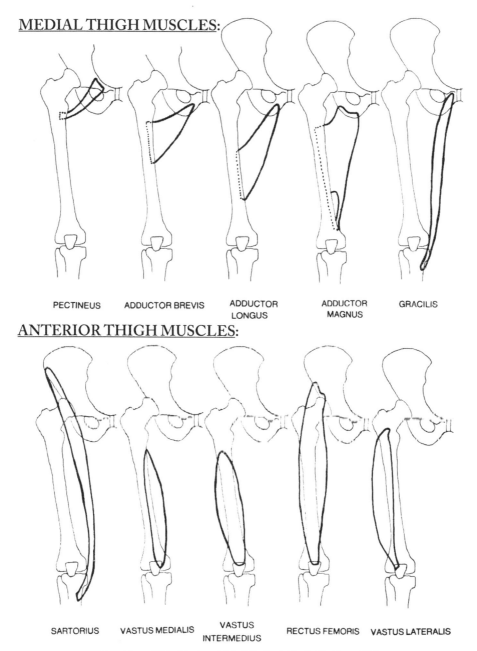

| PECTINEUS | ADDUCTOR BREVIS | ADDUCTOR LONGUS | ADDUCTOR MAGNUS | GRACILIS |

ANTERIOR THIGH MUSCLES:

| SARTORIUS | VASTUS MEDIALIS | VASTUS INTERMEDIUS | RECTUS FEMORIS | VASTUS LATERALIS |

From Goldberg: *Clinical Anatomy Made Ridiculously Simple*, MedMaster, 2007

5.19.) LEG

This chart lists only the <u>main</u> muscle responsible for each movement:

FUNCTION	MAIN MUSCLE	INNERVATION
extension	quadriceps femoris	femoral nerve
flexion	"hamstrings": • semimembranous muscle • semitendinous muscle • biceps femoris	sciatic nerve
inward rotation	semimembranous	sciatic nerve
outward rotation	biceps femoris	sciatic nerve

PULLED HAMSTRINGS:
• Common sports injury in persons who run and kick balls
• Tearing of fibers → very painful

KNEE INJURY:
• Rupture of anterior cruciate ligament: tibia can be drawn anteriorly.
• Rupture of posterior cruciate ligament: tibia can be drawn posteriorly.
• Rupture of lateral ligaments: tibia can be bend laterally.
• Meniscus injuries: pain upon extension of flexed knee (McMurray's test).

The gluteal region is a common side for IM injection of drugs.
- risk of sciatic nerve injury
- upper lateral quadrant is safest

MAIN NERVES OF LEG:

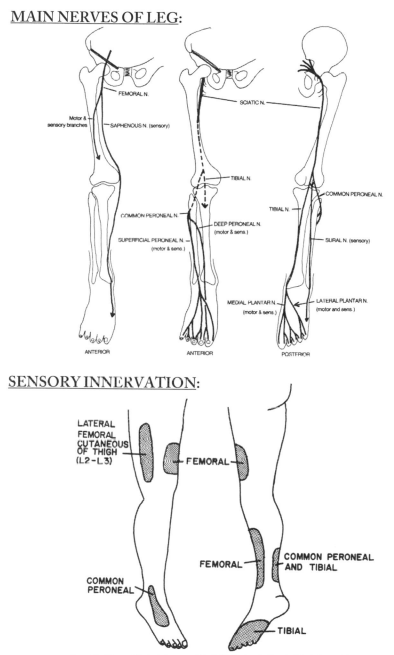

FEMORAL N.

Motor & sensory branches

SAPHENOUS N. (sensory)

SCIATIC N.

TIBIAL N.

COMMON PERONEAL N.

DEEP PERONEAL N. (motor & sens.)

SUPERFICIAL PERONEAL N. (motor & sens.)

TIBIAL N.

COMMON PERONEAL N.

SURAL N. (sensory)

MEDIAL PLANTAR N. (motor & sens.)

LATERAL PLANTAR N. (motor and sens.)

ANTERIOR

ANTERIOR

POSTERIOR

SENSORY INNERVATION:

LATERAL FEMORAL CUTANEOUS OF THIGH (L2-L3)

FEMORAL

FEMORAL

COMMON PERONEAL AND TIBIAL

COMMON PERONEAL

TIBIAL

From Goldberg: *Clinical Anatomy Made Ridiculously Simple*, MedMaster, 2007

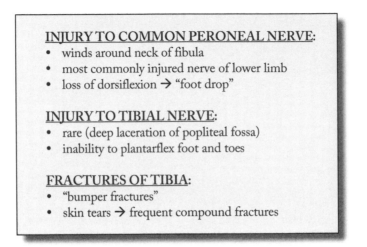

5.20.) FOOT & ANKLE

Notice how each muscle moves the ankle in two axes. Movement in one axis alone requires combined action of two muscles:

MUSCLE	FUNCTION	INNERVATION
tibialis anterior	dorsiflexes + *inverts foot*	deep peroneal nerve
peroneus tertius	dorsiflexes + *everts foot*	deep peroneal nerve
peroneus longus and brevis	plantarflexes + *inverts foot*	superficial peroneal n.
tibialis posterior	plantarflexes + *everts foot*	tibial nerve

PLANTAR FLEXORS

TOE MOVERS

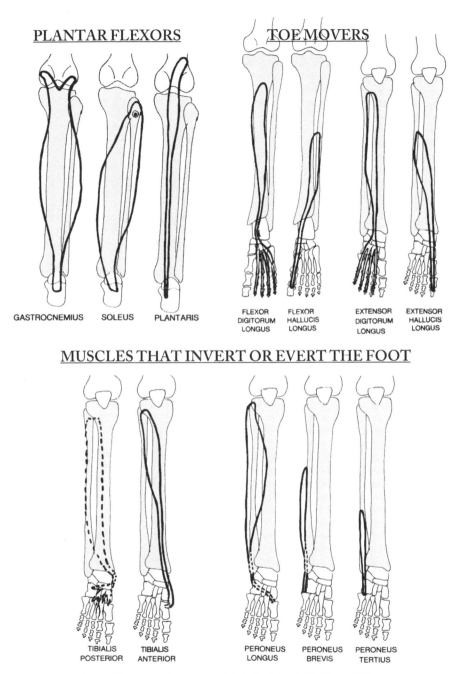

GASTROCNEMIUS SOLEUS PLANTARIS

FLEXOR DIGITORUM LONGUS FLEXOR HALLUCIS LONGUS EXTENSOR DIGITORUM LONGUS EXTENSOR HALLUCIS LONGUS

MUSCLES THAT INVERT OR EVERT THE FOOT

TIBIALIS POSTERIOR TIBIALIS ANTERIOR PERONEUS LONGUS PERONEUS BREVIS PERONEUS TERTIUS

From Goldberg: *Clinical Anatomy Made Ridiculously Simple*, MedMaster, 2007

283

5.21.) <u>MEDIASTINUM</u>

The mediastinum is the space between the lungs (lateral), the sternum (anterior) and the vertebral column (posterior).

A) <u>SUPERIOR MEDIASTINUM</u>:

	CONTENT
superior mediastinum	• thymus • great vessels of heart • trachea • esophagus

B) <u>INFERIOR MEDIASTINUM</u>:

middle mediastinum	• heart
posterior (of heart) mediastinum	• esophagus • descending aorta
anterior (of heart) mediastinum	• large during infancy (filled by thymus) [1]

[1] *in infancy can be wider than the heart silhouette on X-ray!*

5.22.) <u>CORONARY ARTERIES</u>

The heart muscle receives its blood flow from two coronary arteries that originate from the ascending aorta just above the aortic valve.

	SUPPLIES:
left coronary artery → ant. interventricular and circumflex artery	• most of the left atrium • most of the left ventricle • anterior portion of septum
right coronary artery	• right atrium • right ventricle • variable amount of left atrium and ventricle • sinus node • AV node

 Blood flow *through coronary arteries is highest during early diastole and lowest during systole!*

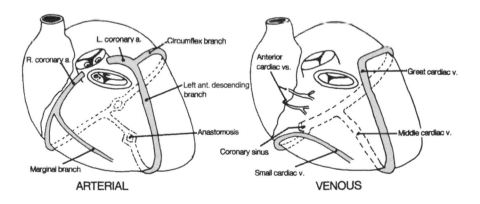

ARTERIAL   VENOUS

From Goldberg: *Clinical Anatomy Made Ridiculously Simple*, MedMaster, 2007

5.23.) ABDOMINAL ARTERIES

Arterial infarctions are rare because these vessels have many anastomoses.
Infarction of the bowels is usually due to interruption of venous drainage.

	BRANCHES	ORGANS
celiac trunk	• left gastric artery • splenic artery • hepatic artery • gastroduodenal artery • sup. pancreaticoduodenal art.	• stomach • spleen • liver • prox. duodenum
sup. mesenteric art.	• inf. pancreaticoduodenal art. many branches	• distal duodenum • small intestine • cecum • ascending colon • transverse colon
inf. mesenteric art.	many branches • superior rectal artery	• descending colon • sigmoid • rectum

---

PORTOCAVAL SHUNTS
gastric/esophageal veins → esophageal varices
anorectal veins → hemorrhoids
paraumbilical veins → caput medusae

5.24.) <u>PERITONEUM</u>

The peritoneum is a serous membrane that covers the entire wall and wraps over the viscera contained in it. In men, it forms a closed sac. In women, it is pierced by the uterine tubes.

INTRAPERITONEAL	RETROPERITONEAL
• stomach • small bowel • transverse colon • spleen ○ part of liver	• aorta • vena cava • kidneys • pancreas • duodenum • ascending colon • descending colon

<u>ACUTE APPENDICITIS</u>
McBurney's point: at junction between lateral and middle
thirds of a line between umbilicus and
anterior superior iliac spine.

<u>Signs of peritonitis</u>:
• *severe pain (localized or diffuse)*
• *rebound tenderness*
• *abdominal muscle rigidity*

5.25.) <u>LAYERS OF SPERMATIC CORD</u>

Since the inguinal canal is formed by the descending testis, it is easy to see how the layers of the spermatic cord are derived from the layers of the abdominal wall:

deep

loose connective tissue	arteries, pampiniform plexus
internal spermatic fascia	from fascia transversalis
cremaster muscle and fascia	from int. oblique muscle
external spermatic fascia	from ext. oblique aponeurosis
superficial fascia	contains dartos muscle

superficial

5.26.) <u>OVARY / TESTIS</u>

"Important organs receive multiple blood supplies":

ovary	• aorta → ovarian artery • internal iliac art. → uterine artery
testis	• aorta → testicular artery • internal iliac art. → art. of ductus deferens • inf. epigastric art. → cremasteric artery

MUSCLES FORMING THE INGUINAL CANAL:

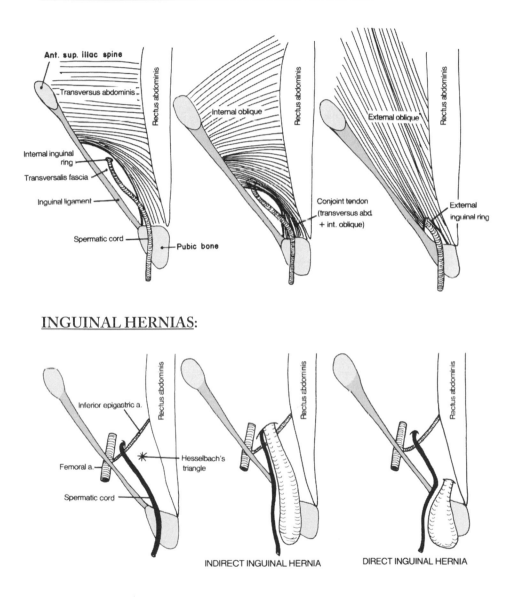

INGUINAL HERNIAS:

From Goldberg: *Clinical Anatomy Made Ridiculously Simple*, MedMaster, 2007

Part C : Neuroanatomy

5.27.) CORTEX

The two hemispheres are connected by the corpus callosum. Patients with complete transection of the corpus have subtle cognitive deficits relating verbal expression of non-verbal input:

LEFT HEMISPHERE	RIGHT HEMISPHERE
• language	• non-verbal
• mathematics	• musical
• sequential	• geometrical
• analytical	• spatial comprehension

vision	occipital lobe
hearing	temporal lobe
taste	insula, below postcentral gyrus
reading, writing	angular gyrus
primary motor cortex	precentral gyrus
primary sensory cortex	postcentral gyrus
Wernicke (sensory)	temporal lobe, superior gyrus
Broca (motor)	frontal lobe, near lateral fissure

APHASIAS
Broca: nonfluent speech, good comprehension
Wernicke: fluent but nonsensical speech, poor comprehension

5.28.) CEREBRAL ARTERIES

Stroke: 80% ischemic, 20% hemorrhagic

The circle of Willis receives blood supply from the 2 carotid arteries and the basilar artery. It gives rise to 3 pairs of cerebral arteries:

	SUPPLIES:	OCCLUSION RESULTS IN:
ant. cerebral a.	medial cortex	motor & sensory loss (contralateral legs and feet)
middle cerebral a.	lateral cortex ant. limb of int. capsule	motor & sensory loss (contralateral upper body)
post. cerebral a.	occipital cortex	homonymous hemianopsia (contralateral)
ant. choroidal a.	basal ganglia hypothalamus post. limb of internal capsule	
cerebellar aa.	cerebellum lateral portions of brain stem	ataxia brainstem syndromes

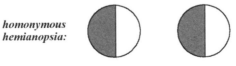

homonymous hemianopsia:

left   right

BLOOD SUPPLY OF CORTEX:

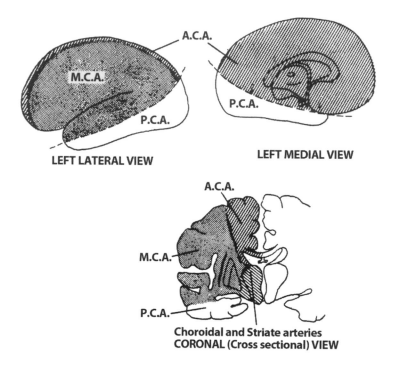

LEFT LATERAL VIEW

LEFT MEDIAL VIEW

Choroidal and Striate arteries
CORONAL (Cross sectional) VIEW

From Goldberg: *Clinical Neuroanatomy Made Ridiculously Simple*, MedMaster, 2007

A.C.A = anterior cerebral artery
M.C.A = middle cerebral artery
P.C.A = posterior cerebral artery

5.29.) TRANSIENT ISCHEMIC ATTACKS

TIAs are caused by <u>partial</u> occlusion of cerebral arteries by plaques or emboli. They may be precursors to a full stroke and it is important to recognize the symptoms:

INTERNAL CAROTID ARTERY	VERTEBROBASILAR ART.
o ipsilateral monocular blindness ("amaurosis fugax") o hemiparesis, contralateral o hemisensory loss, contralateral o language disturbance	o vertigo o diplopia o ataxia o facial numbness/weakness o nausea

5.30.) HYPERTENSIVE HEMORRHAGE

HEMORRHAGE INTO:	RESULTS IN:
putamen	• contralateral weakness, including face • contralateral hemianopsia
thalamus	• contralateral hemiparesis • sensory changes • homonymous hemianopsia
pons	• coma • small reactive pupils • quadriplegia
cerebellum	• unsteady gait • clumsiness • nausea, vomiting

5.31.) CRANIAL NERVES

Most cranial nerves carry both motor and sensory functions. Visceral motor nerves form the "autonomic nervous system".

A) MOTOR:

	NERVE	FUNCTIONS
somatic motor	III	• extraocular eye muscles (except sup. oblique and lat. rectus)
	IV	• superior oblique
	VI	• lateral rectus
	XII	• tongue muscles (except palatoglossus)
branchial motor (derived from branchial arches)	V	• mastication
	VII	• facial expression
	IX, X	• pharynx, larynx
	XI	• trapezius, sternocleidomastoid muscles
visceral motor	III	• ciliary muscle, constrictor pupillae
	VII	• all glands except parotid
	IX	• parotid
	X	• abdominal viscera up to splenic flexure

B) SENSORY:

special sensory	I	• smell
	II	• vision
	VII, IX	• taste
	VIII	• hearing, balance
general sensory	V, VII, IX, X	• pain, temperature, touch, proprioception
visceral sensory	IX, X	• afferents for visceral reflexes

5.32.) <u>VISUAL SYSTEM</u>

Lesions in the optical tract cause very characteristic deficits in the visual field. Try not to memorize only, but try to understand why exactly these defects occur.

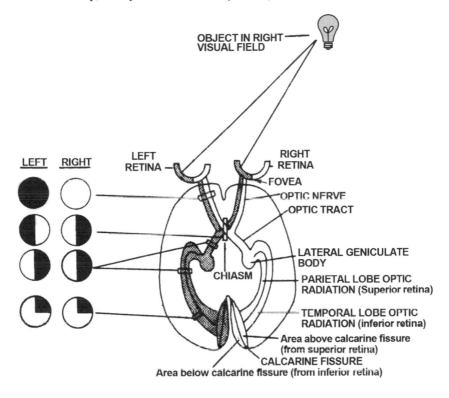

Modified from Goldberg: *Clinical Neuroanatomy Made Ridiculously Simple*, MedMaster, 2007

Notice, how objects in the RIGHT visual field are represented in the LEFT portion of both left and right retinas.

5.33.) PARASYMPATHETIC GANGLIA

The parasympathetic nervous system has a cranial and a sacral component. No parasympathetic fibers originate in the cervical, thoracic or lumbar segments. This chart summarizes the functions of the cranial portion of the parasympathetic nervous system:

NUCLEUS	NERVE	GANGLION	ORGANS
Edinger-Westphal	III	ciliary	eye
sup. salivary nucleus	VII	sublingual submaxillary	lacrimal gland nasal glands submandibular gland
inf. salivary nucleus	IX	otic	parotid gland
dorsal motor nucleus	X	many, mostly intramural	many

Pupillary light reflex: *Optical nerve → tectal area → Edinger-Westphal nucleus → parasympathetic → sphincter*
Argyll-Robertson pupil: *Damage to tectal area (e.g. syphilis): pupils constrict for near vision but not for light.*

5.34.) __BASAL GANGLIA__

The basal ganglia receive input from all parts of the cortex and also project via the thalamus to the precentral motor cortex. They are involved in the programming of movement.

striatum	• caudate • putamen • globus pallidus
neostriatum	• caudate • putamen
paleostriatum	• globus pallidus
lentiform nucleus	• putamen • globus pallidus

PARKINSON'S DISEASE
- loss of dopaminergic input from substantia nigra to striatum
o bradykinesia (difficulty initiating or stopping a movement)
o muscle rigidity
o tremor ("pill-rolling")

HUNTINGTON'S DISEASE
- atrophy of caudate nucleus
o chorea: involuntary movements
o personality changes, dementia

WILSON'S DISEASE
- copper accumulation in lentiform nucleus (and elsewhere)
o tremor, spasticity, chorea, bizarre behavior

5.35.) THALAMUS

"Thalamus knows all" (receives all sensory input, except olfactory) !!!

The thalamus is the major sensory relay station of the brain. Thalamic-cortical interactions also determine consciousness and the sleep/wake cycle.

I.) ANTERIOR THALAMUS (part of limbic system)	input: mammillary bodies output: cingula (cortex)
II.) LATERAL THALAMUS	major nucleus: "pulvinar"
ventral anterior nucleus	receives input from basal ganglia output to premotor cortex
ventral posterior nucleus	**VPL:** medial lemniscus, spinothalamic tract (proprioception, touch) **VPM:** trigeminal nerve (taste)
ventrolateral nucleus	input from cerebellum and basal ganglia output to motor cortex
III.) MEDIAL THALAMUS	projects to frontal cortex
IV.) POSTERIOR THALAMUS	**medial geniculate:** auditory pathway **lateral geniculate:** optic tract

> **General Features of Thalamus:**
> - major synaptic relay station (sensory input)
> - basal ganglia → thalamus → cortex
> - rhythm established by thalamus forms major contribution to EEG

Some patients with thalamic injury become insensitive to pain and other sensory stimuli.

5.36.) BRAINSTEM SYNDROMES

Brainstem syndromes are complex because many structures are packed tightly together in a small space. The most famous one is the <u>Wallenberg syndrome</u> (lateral medulla infarction due to occlusion of posterior inferior cerebellar artery).

	BLOOD SUPPLY
medulla	**lateral:** posterior inferior cerebellar artery **medial:** anterior spinal artery
lower pons	**lateral:** anterior inferior cerebellar artery **medial:** basilar artery
upper pons	**lateral:** superior cerebellar artery **medial:** basilar artery

The brainstem contains vital centers (respiratory and cardiovascular) and the reticular activating system that projects to the thalamus and determines consciousness. A crude way to assess brainstem function in your patients is to check their pupillary light reflex.

5.37.) <u>MEDULLA</u>

Infarction of lateral medulla: = Wallenberg

DAMAGE TO:	RESULTS IN:
spinal tract nucleus V	ipsilateral face: pain / temp loss
nucleus solitarius	ipsilateral tongue: loss of taste
reticular formation	ipsilateral Horner's syndrome
nucleus ambiguus	hoarseness loss of pharyngeal reflex
spinothalamic tract	contralateral body pain / temp loss

Infarction of medial medulla:

DAMAGE TO:	RESULTS IN:
hypoglossal muscle	ipsilateral tongue: atrophic paralysis
medial lemniscus	contralateral loss of position sense contralateral loss of vibration sense
pyramidal tract	contralateral body: spastic paralysis

5.38.) <u>LOWER PONS</u>

Infarction of lateral pons:

DAMAGE TO:	RESULTS IN:
spinocerebellar tract	ipsilateral limb ataxia
nucleus VII	ipsilateral face: paralysis
spinal tract nucleus V	ipsilateral face: loss of sensation
reticular formation	ipsilateral Horner's syndrome
vestibular nucleus	vertigo
cochlear nuclei	deafness / tinnitus

Infarction of medial pons:

DAMAGE TO:	RESULTS IN:
nucleus VII	ipsilateral face: spastic paralysis
medial long. fasciculus	ipsilateral eye can not adduct on lateral gaze
nucleus VI	ipsilateral paralysis of lat. rectus oculi
corticospinal tract	contralateral body: spastic paralysis
medial lemniscus	contralateral loss of position and vibration sense

5.39.) UPPER PONS

Infarction of lateral pons:

DAMAGE TO:	RESULTS IN:
motor nucleus V	ipsilateral loss of masseter function
reticular formation	ipsilateral Horner's syndrome
spinothalamic tract	contralateral loss of pain and sensation

Infarction of medial pons:

DAMAGE TO:	RESULTS IN:
corticospinal tract	contralateral spastic paralysis

A. Superior colliculus / Aqueduct / Medial geniculate body / Red nucleus / Substantia nigra / Corticospinal tract

B. Inferior colliculus / Aqueduct / Decussation of superior cerebellar peduncles / Substantia nigra / Corticospinal tract

C. Corticospinal tract (broken up) — 4th Vent

A upper midbrain
B lower midbrain
C pons
D upper medulla
E lower medulla

D. 4th Ventricle / Inferior olive / Corticospinal tract

E. Nucleus gracilis / Nucleus cuneatus / Spinal tract and nucleus of CN5 / Decussation of medial lemniscus / Decussation of corticospinal tract

From Goldberg: *Clinical Neuroanatomy Made Ridiculously Simple*, MedMaster, 2007

5.40.) <u>CROSSING OVER SITES</u>

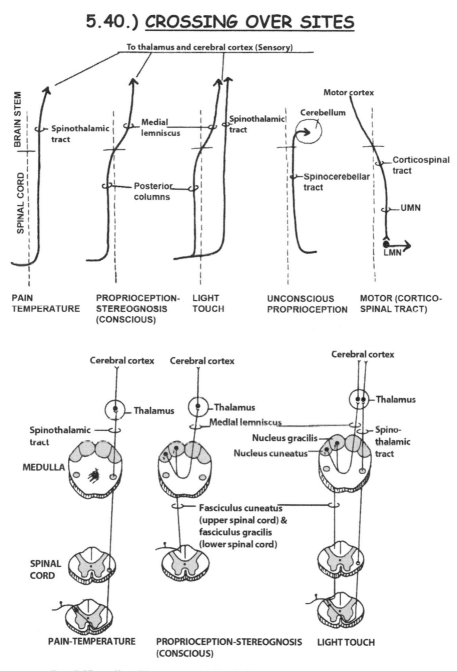

From Goldberg: *Clinical Neuroanatomy Made Ridiculously Simple*, MedMaster, 2007

5.41.) WHERE IS THE LESION?

A large part of neurology is to localize the lesion based on your knowledge of neuroanatomy:

TYPICAL SYMPTOMS	LESION
Loss of pain and temperature sensation arms and shoulder	Syringomyelia
Muscle weakness and loss of sensation in left arm	Right middle cerebral a.
Muscle weakness and loss of sensation in left leg	Right anterior cerebral a.
Spastic paralysis, loss of proprioception left leg and loss of pain and temperature sensation right leg	Hemisection of left spinal cord
Spastic paralysis both legs	Total transection of spinal cord
Flaccid paralysis, loss of sensations, both legs	Guillain-Barré syndrome
Muscle atrophy, fasciculations both arms & legs	ALS
Loss of pain and temperature sensation left arms, legs, body Paralysis of left arms, legs and body Loss of sensation right lower face	"Wallenberg syndrome" (right lateral medulla)
Sensory loss both hands and feet ("sock & glove pattern")	Peripheral neuropathy
Loss of sensation over buttocks, perineum and impotence	Cauda equina lesion

5.42.) <u>KEY DERMATOMES</u>

skull	C2
thumb	C6
nipple	T5
belly button	T10
big toe	L4
penis	S3
anus	S5
knee jerk reflex	**L4**
ankle jerk reflex	**S1**

 The lowest segment (S5) is around the anus, not the toes!

PHYSIOLOGY

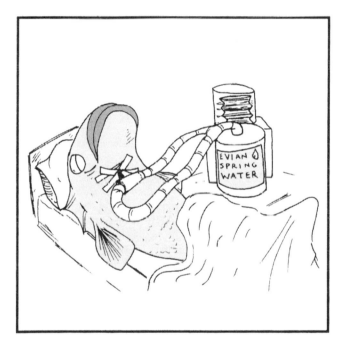

Fish Respirators.

6.1.) SIX EQUATIONS YOU REALLY NEED

1. HOW TO CALCULATE TOTAL PERIPHERAL RESISTANCE:

Mean blood pressure $P_{average} = P_{diastolic} + 1/3 \, (P_{systolic} - P_{diastolic})$

Total peripheral resistance   TPR = mean blood pressure / cardiac output

EXAMPLE: systolic blood pressure 120 mmHg
diastolic blood pressure 80 mmHg
cardiac output 5,000 ml/min

→ mean pressure = 80 +1/3 (120-80) = 93 mmHg
→ TPR = 93/5,000 = 0.018

Norepinephrine increases TPR (α-receptors → vasoconstriction)
Epinephrine decreases TPR (β-receptors → vasodilation)

2. HOW TO CALCULATE CARDIAC OUTPUT:

Cardiac output = systemic blood flow = pulmonary blood flow
(Assuming that there are no intracardiac shunts!)

Fick's Principle: pulmonary flow = oxygen uptake / (a-v oxygen difference)

EXAMPLE: arterial O_2 = 20 ml oxygen / 100 ml blood = 0.2
venous O_2 = 15 ml oxygen / 100 ml blood = 0.15
oxygen uptake = 250 ml / min

→ cardiac output = 250 / 0.05 = 5,000 ml / min

Cardiac output is usually normalized to body surface area (= "cardiac index").

3. HOW TO CALCULATE RENAL CLEARANCE:

Clearance of X   clearance $\cdot$ $[X]_{plasma}$ = urine flow $\cdot$ $[X]_{urine}$

EXAMPLE: plasma creatinine concentration = 1.5 mg/dl
urine creatinine concentration = 180 mg/dl
urine flow = 1,500 ml / 24 h $\approx$ 1 ml/min

→ creatinine clearance = 1 ml/min (180/1.5) = 120 ml/min

4. ACID / BASE CALCULATIONS:

Henderson-Hasselbalch $pH = pK + \log \dfrac{[salt]}{[acid]}$

$$pH = 6.1 + \log \frac{[HCO_3^-]}{[CO_2]}$$

$$pH = 6.1 + \log \frac{[HCO_3^-]}{0.03\, PCO_2}$$

EXAMPLE: plasma bicarbonate = 24 mM/l
PCO_2 = 40 mmHg

→ pH = 6.1 + log (24/1.2) = 6.1 + log (20) = 7.4

*Bicarbonate is a powerful buffer (despite having a pK 6.1 far from physiological
pH) because the acid (H_2CO_3 ↔ CO_2) and salt (HCO_3^-) concentrations are
independently regulated by the body:*
- *Kidneys regulate HCO_3^-*
- *Lung ventilation regulates CO_2*

---

log 0.1 = -1   /   log 1 = 0   /   log 10 = 1   /   log 100 = 2   etc....

---

5. HOW TO CALCULATE DIFFUSION CAPACITY OF THE LUNG:

Diffusion (Fick's law) $\text{flow} = D \cdot \text{area} \cdot \dfrac{\text{concentration gradient}}{\text{membrane thickness}}$

Since lung area and membrane thickness of the lung cannot be measured directly, they are lumped together with the diffusion coefficient:

$$\text{flow} = DL \cdot \text{concentration gradient}$$

EXAMPLE: alveolar partial pressure of CO = 200 mmHg
blood partial pressure of CO = 0 mmHg
flow = 4,000 ml/min

→ CO diffusion capacity DL_{CO} = 20 ml / min · mmHg

CO_2 and O_2 equilibrate within $1/3^{rd}$ of capillary transient time (perfusion limited!)

CO on the other hand is less lipid soluble (diffusion limited) and therefore well suited for measuring diffusion properties of the lung. This is done with a single inspiration of diluted CO and measuring the rate of disappearance of CO from alveolar gas.

Increased DL: Recruitment and dilation of pulmonary capillaries.
(may double during exercise!)

Decreased DL: Interstitial lung diseases, emphysema and V/Q imbalance.

6. HOW TO CALCULATE LUNG COMPLIANCE:

Elasticity $\text{elasticity} = \dfrac{\Delta \text{ pressure}}{\Delta \text{ volume}}$

Compliance (="stretchability") $\text{compliance} = 1/\text{elasticity} = \dfrac{\Delta \text{ volume}}{\Delta \text{ pressure}}$

Patient's with COPD have lungs with __high__ compliance.
Patient's with restrictive lung disease have __low__ compliance.
A rod of steal has higher elasticity (less stretchability) than a rubber band.

6.2.) <u>ION CHANNELS</u>

Ion channels are most crucial for excitatory cells. Opening of these channels results in membrane potential moving towards the equilibrium potential for [X]. You can calculate the equilibrium potential of [X] from intracellular and extracellular [X] concentrations (Nernst equation).

	KEY FEATURES
K^+ channels	• maintain resting membrane potential • repolarization phase of action potentials • afterhyperpolarization
Na^+ channels	• upstroke phase of neuronal action potential • phase 0 of cardiac action potential (myocyte) • rapid inactivation → repolarization (refractory period)
Ca^{2+} channels	• excitation-contraction coupling • excitation-secretion coupling • phase 0 of cardiac pacemaker cells (sinus node) • cardiac plateau phase: Ca^{2+} entry • intracellular Ca^{2+} release (ryanodine receptor)
cation channels	• depolarization • dark current of photoreceptors • nicotinic ACh receptor at motor endplate
Cl^- channels	• CNS: inhibitory postsynaptic potentials
Na^+ / K^+ pump	• maintains ion gradients • is electrogenic: 3 Na^+ out for 2 K^+ in (but direct contribution to RMP is very small)

<u>Absolute refractory period</u>:
Action potentials cannot be generated because of inactivation of the Na^+ channels.
<u>Relative refractory period</u>:
Some Na^+ channels have recovered from inactivation. Strong stimuli may generate action potentials with slow upstroke and low amplitude.

6.3.) TRANSPORT

Lipid bilayers are permeable for water (!) and small, uncharged molecules. Other molecules require membrane transport proteins, either **carriers** which take advantage of concentration gradients or **pumps** which derive their energy from ATP.

	PASSIVE (diffusion)	**FACILITATED** (carriers)	**ACTIVE** (pumps)
		TRANSPORTERS	
ATP required?	no	no	yes
can transport against gradient?	no	no (yes if coupled)	yes
substrate specific?	no	yes	yes
saturating?	no	yes	yes

EXAMPLES:

- **Active transport:** Na^+ / K^+ ATPase
                              H^+ / K^+ ATPase

- **Facilitated transport:**   simple glucose carriers

  Secondary active transport: Na^+ / glucose carriers
                              Na^+ / amino acid carriers
  (Glucose and amino acids are transported <u>against</u> their gradients, but this is driven by Na^+ moving down its own gradient.)

- **Passive transport:**   water, electrolytes, O_2 etc.

6.4.) <u>SIGNAL TRANSDUCTION</u>

2nd messengers are generated intracellularly and amplify the signal:
- receptor → G protein → adenylyl cyclase → cAMP → protein kinase A
- nitric oxide → guanylyl cyclase → cGMP → protein kinase G
- receptor → G protein → phospholipase C → IP3, DAG → protein kinase C

	HORMONES / RECEPTORS
cAMP ↑	• β, H2 receptors • ACTH
cAMP ↓	• α2 receptors • M2, M4 receptors
cGMP ↑	• nitric oxide • ANP • Viagra ™ 1
IP3, DAG	• α1, M1, M3, H1 receptors • angiotensin receptors • tachykinins • endothelin
tyrosine kinase	• insulin • growth factors
gene expression	• steroid hormones • thyroid hormones • retinoic acid

[1] *inhibits type V cGMP phosphodiesterase → enhanced effect of nitric oxide on penile artery dilation.*

__Tyrosine kinase__ phosphorylates many proteins. It also activates the ras → raf → MAP kinase cascade which modulates gene expression. Out of control activation of ras is a/w with many neoplasms.

G proteins work like a timer mechanism:

- Hormone receptor interaction first sets the timer (GDP on α-subunit is replaced by GTP), then starts it (α-subunit dissociates from β/γ).
- Activated α-subunit interacts with other enzymes such as adenylyl cyclase.
- α-subunit has built-in enzymatic activity that hydrolyzes its GTP to GDP, which terminates the action of the α-subunit ("time is up").

Gi	inhibits adenylate cyclase
Gs	stimulates adenylate cyclase
Gq	activates phospholipase C

6.5.) NERVE FIBERS

large diameter
high velocity

Aα	• efferent: skeletal muscle • afferent: from muscle spindle
Aγ	• efferent: to muscle spindle
Aβ , Aδ	• afferent: touch fast sharp pain
C	• afferent: slow dull pain
B , C	• efferent: autonomic nerves

small diameter
low velocity

"All-or-None" response:

If the stimulus is not strong enough to depolarize the membrane to threshold, no action potential occurs. If threshold is reached, a uniform action potential is generated. Stimulus strength determines frequency but not amplitude of action potentials.

6.6.) <u>TOUCH RECEPTORS</u>

Specialized receptors mediate the five sensory modalities:

A) <u>SENSORY FIBERS TRAVELLING IN DORSAL COLUMNS</u>:

1. pressure	• Merkel cells *(slowly adapting)*
2. light touch	• Meissner's corpuscle *(fast adapting)* • hair follicle sensors
3. vibration	• Pacinian corpuscle *(most rapidly adapting)*

B) <u>SENSORY FIBERS TRAVELLING IN SPINOTHALAMIC TRACT</u>:

4. pain	• mostly free nerve endings
5. temperature	• mostly free nerve endings

Paradoxical cold: *At temperatures > 45°C (120F) cold fibers begin to fire again (together with pain fibers). This sensation of pain and coolness is called "paradoxical cold".*

6.7.) <u>ACCOMMODATION</u>

Accommodation adjusts the lens to the distance of the object, to obtain an in-focus image on the retina. In addition, the pupils constrict when focusing a near object ("accommodation reflex").

NEAR OBJECT	FAR OBJECT
ciliary muscle contracted	ciliary muscle relaxed
zonula fibers relaxed	zonula fibers tense
lens rounded (if elastic)	lens flat
focal length short	focal length far

myopia (nearsightedness)	• lens has normal elasticity • focal point too short (or eye ball too long) *corrected with negative lens (concave)*
hypermetropia (farsightedness)	• lens has normal elasticity • focal point too far (or eye ball too short) *corrected with positive lens (convex)*
presbyopia (age)	• lens has lost elasticity • cannot shorten focal length *corrected with positive lens (convex)*

 Patients with hypermetropia or presbyopia have difficulty reading.

316

6.8.) NYSTAGMUS

Involuntary rhythmic movements of eyes, usually horizontal, that have a slow phase followed by a rapid snap back. Direction of nystagmus is defined by the fast phase.

optokinetic	• looking out of train *nystagmus against movement of image*
vestibular	• postrotational nystagmus *nystagmus against direction of prior rotation* • caloric nystagmus *nystagmus away from cold ear*
pathologic	**horizontal:** vestibular disease **vertical:** brainstem disease

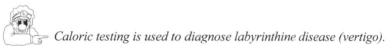

Caloric testing is used to diagnose labyrinthine disease (vertigo).

6.9.) COCHLEA

The endocochlear potential is +80 mV, as a result, hair cells have a membrane potential of −150 mV relative to scala media, making them very sensitive to permeability changes.

scala vestibuli	Na$^+$ rich	perilymph
scala media	K$^+$ rich	endolymph
scala tympani	Na$^+$ rich	perilymph

> **pitch:** frequency range 20-20,000 Hz
> **loudness:** pressure range 0-140 dB
>
> 10 dB = 10 fold change in sound intensity
> 20 dB = 100 fold change in sound intensity

6.10.) <u>DEAFNESS</u>

In patients with diminished hearing it is important to distinguish between middle ear from inner ear problems. This can be done with a simple tuning fork test:

TUNING FORK TESTS:

	WEBER	RINNE
method	Place fork on top of skull	Place fork on mastoid process until tone disappears (= bone conduction). Then hold next to ear (= air conduction).
normal	Sound is equal in both ears.	Air conduction is better than bone conduction.
conduction deafness [1] (middle ear)	Sound lateralized to sick ear.	Bone conduction is better than air conduction.
nerve deafness [2] (inner ear)	Sound lateralized to normal ear.	Air conduction is better than bone conduction.

[1] *chronic otitis, otosclerosis or occlusion of external auditory meatus*
[2] *cochlear disease or injury to cranial nerve VIII.*

Unilateral cortical lesions do NOT affect hearing since cochlear nuclei project to both temporal lobes.

6.11.) <u>AUTONOMIC NERVOUS SYSTEM</u>

The ANS has 3 major divisions (1.) enteric, (2.) sympathetic and (3.) parasympathetic.
The sympathetic nervous system mediates the *"flight or fright"* response, while the parasympathetic
nervous system has several discrete functions: digestion, micturition, erection, pupillary light reflex...

	SYMPATHETIC	PARASYMPATHETIC
heart	• increased heart rate • increased conduction • increased contraction	• decreased heart rate
bronchi	• dilates	• constricts
GI tract	• reduces motility	• increases motility
sphincters of GI	• constricts	• relaxes
rectum	• allows filling	• empties • relaxes internal sphincter
bladder	• allows filling	• empties • relaxes internal sphincter
erection		• erection
ejaculation	• triggers ejaculation	
pupils of eye	• big (mydriasis)	• small (miosis)
sweat glands	• sweat (cholinergic!)	
salivary glands		• secretion

blood vessels	• depends on receptors:
	  - α constricts
	  - β dilates
		• dilates artery of penis
		only

> ### <u>4 ways to decrease blood pressure:</u>
> 1. block nicotinic ganglionic receptors
> 2. block β receptors
> 3. block α1 receptors
> 4. stimulate α2 receptors

6.12.) <u>CHOLINERGIC RECEPTORS</u>

There are 2 classes of cholinergic receptors (1.) nicotinic receptors stimulated by nicotine and (2.) muscarinic receptors stimulated by muscarine.

	LOCATION
nicotinic	• **autonomic ganglia** • **sympathetic and parasympathetic ganglia!** • **adrenal medulla** • **neuromuscular junction** these receptors differ from autonomic ones! SIGNAL TRANSDUCTION ligand-gated non-selective cation channel
muscarinic	• **postsynaptic parasympathetic** • **sweat glands** (innervated by sympathetic nerves!) SIGNAL TRANSDUCTION *second messenger depends on receptor subtype:* M1, M3 → PLC → IP3, DAG M2, M4 → inhibit adenylate cyclase → cAMP↓

Antagonists: Nicotinic (ganglionic):   hexamethonium
Nicotinic (motor endplate):   tubocurarine
Muscarinic: atropine

Sympathetic   ACh (nicotinic)   Norepinephrine (adrenergic)

Parasympathetic   ACh (nicotinic)   ACh (muscarinic)

Somatic Motor   ACh (nicotinic)

From Olson: *Clinical Pharmacology Made Ridiculously Simple*, MedMaster, 2007

6.13.) <u>ADRENERGIC RECEPTORS</u>

There are 2 classes of adrenergic receptors (1.) α-receptors, which are excitatory except in the GI tract and (2.) β-receptors, which are inhibitory except at the heart.

alpha-1	• **postsynaptic sympathetic** • generally excitatory (vasoconstriction) • in GI tract inhibitory *Gq → phospholipase C → IP3, DAG*
alpha-2	• **presynaptic sympathetic** (decrease catecholamine release) • **central nervous system** (decrease sympathetic tone) *Gi → inhibits adenylate cyclase → cAMP↓*
beta-1	• **postsynaptic sympathetic (cardiac)** excitatory (chronotrope, dromotrope, inotrope) *Gs → adenylate cyclase → cAMP↑*
beta-2	• **postsynaptic sympathetic (all others)** inhibitory (vasodilation, bronchodilation) *Gs → adenylate cyclase → cAMP↑*

Agonists: ***alpha:*** *epinephrine ≥ norepinephrine >> isoproterenol*
beta 1 : *isoproterenol > epinephrine = norepinephrine*
beta 2 : *isoproterenol > epinephrine >> norepinephrine*

<u>Vascular tone:</u>
Norepinephrine injection → stimulates α-receptors → vasoconstriction → increase in diastolic blood pressure.

Epinephrine injection → stimulates α and β-receptors, but β-effect predominates → vasodilation → decrease in diastolic blood pressure.

6.14.) CONTROL OF HEART BEAT

The heart receives tonic input from both sympathetic and parasympathetic nerves and the heart rate depends on the balance of the two. In humans, parasympathetic tone is stronger → removal of both sympathetic and parasympathetic innervation results in increased heart rate!

right vagus nerve	• slows frequency (sinus node)
left vagus nerve	• slows conduction (AV node) • decreased force of contraction (atria but not ventricles!)
sympathetic	• increased frequency • increased conduction • increased force of contraction (atria and ventricles)
epinephrine injection	• increased conduction and contraction • increased frequency • *increased systolic pressure* • *decreased diastolic pressure (vasodilation)*
norepinephrine injection	• increased conduction and contraction • decreased frequency (baroreceptor reflex !) • *increased systolic pressure* • *increased diastolic pressure (vasoconstriction)*

> ### Frank-Starling mechanism:
> Preload = end-diastolic volume in ventricle
> Preload↑ → muscle filament overlap↑ → stroke volume↑

6.15.) <u>SKELETAL MUSCLE</u>

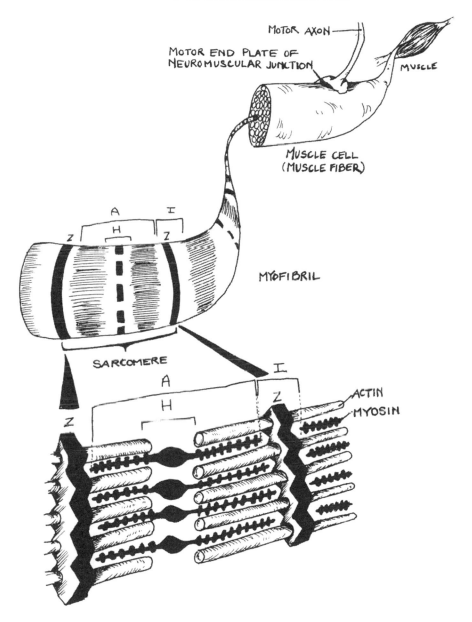

MOTOR AXON

MOTOR END PLATE OF
NEUROMUSCULAR JUNCTION

MUSCLE

MUSCLE CELL
(MUSCLE FIBER)

A

I

H

Z

Z

MYOFIBRIL

SARCOMERE

A

I

H

Z

Z

ACTIN

MYOSIN

From Goldberg: *Clinical Physiology Made Ridiculously Simple*, MedMaster, 2007

6.16.) <u>CONTROL OF MUSCLE TONE</u>

Muscle tone is "fine-tuned" by two sensory organs:

	FUNCTION	NERVE FIBER
muscle spindle	• measures muscle length • activates α-motoneuron when stretched	γ efferent 1A afferent
Golgi tendon organ	• measures muscle tension • inhibits α-motoneuron	1B afferent

STRETCH REFLEX (example: knee jerk reflex): *Intrafusal fibers (muscle spindle) run parallel with skeletal muscle fibers. Stretching results in firing of 1A afferents that excite the α-motoneuron (monosynaptic reflex). The α-motoneuron of the antagonistic muscle is inhibited via an interneuron.*

<u>Increased muscle tone</u>:
- activation of γ-fibers
- upper motor neuron lesions (hemiplegia)
- Parkinson
- cold, anxiety

<u>Decreased muscle tone</u>:
- lower motor neuron lesions
- spinal shock (early phase of hemiplegia)
- warmth

<u>Decorticate posture</u>:
- legs extended, arms flexed (cortex injury)

<u>Decerebrate posture</u>:
- legs and arms extended (brainstem injury)

6.17.) MUSCLE TYPES

"Fast" muscles are for rapid, powerful actions (jumping, short distance running) while "slow" muscles are for prolonged activity (body posture, marathon).

	RED SKELETAL MUSCLE	WHITE SKELETAL MUSCLE
myosin isoenzyme	slow	fast
glycolytic capacity	low	high
oxidative capacity	high	low

related to:
• number of capillaries
• myoglobin content
• number of mitochondria

isotonic: force remains constant
muscle shortens during contraction

isometric: force increases during contraction
length of muscle remains constant

6.18.) <u>ELECTROMECHANICAL COUPLING</u>

Electromechanical coupling describes the relationship between membrane potential, intracellular Ca^{2+} and muscle contraction. There are important differences between the 3 muscle tissues:

SKELETAL MUSCLE	HEART MUSCLE	SMOOTH MUSCLE
motor units [1]	syncytium	syncytium
action potential: 2-4 ms	action potential: 200-400 ms	<u>tonic</u> • vascular smooth muscle <u>phasic</u> • visceral smooth muscle • slow waves, spikes
Ca^{2+} binds to troponin	Ca^{2+} binds to troponin	Ca^{2+} -calmodulin → MLC phosphorylation
Ca^{2+} release from SR	Ca^{2+} influx	Ca^{2+} influx and release
tetanus	no tetanus	myogenic tone

[1] *motor unit = all the muscle fibers that are innervated by one α-motoneuron*

<u>REGULATION OF STRENGTH</u>:

SKELETAL MUSCLE	HEART MUSCLE	SMOOTH MUSCLE
• recruitment of motor units • AP frequency	• AP duration	• membrane potential • biochemical modulation of Ca^{2+} sensitivity

6.19.) <u>CARDIAC CYCLE</u>

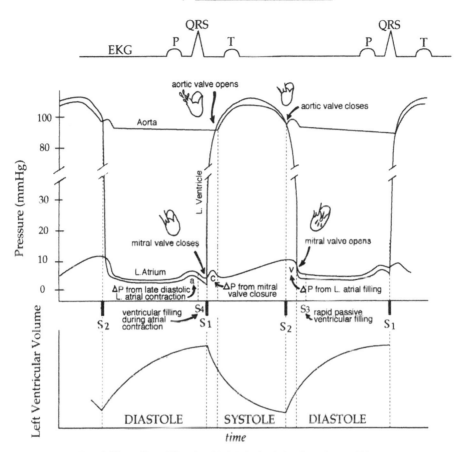

From Goldberg: *Clinical Physiology Made Ridiculously Simple*, MedMaster, 2007

a-wave : atrial contraction   **c-wave** : bulging of mitral valve
v-wave : filling of atria

All valves are closed during isovolumetric contraction or relaxation.

6.20.) <u>LUNG VOLUMES</u>

Lung volumes are important for diagnosis and need to be monitored in patients with restrictive or obstructive lung diseases.

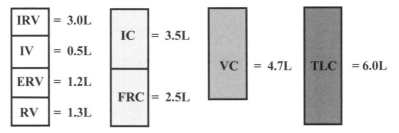

- IRV, IV and ERV are measured by spirometer
- RV is measured by helium dilution or body plethysmography

Ventilation = dV/dt
Alveolar ventilation = ventilation - dead space ventilation

- **Dead space is measured by nitrogen exhalation**
  (inhale 100% oxygen, measure N_2 while exhaling)

Dead space = anatomical dead space plus unperfused alveoli
Ventilated alveoli that are unperfused (for example pulmonary embolism) increase dead space. This situation is called V/Q mismatch.

> <u>Ventilation / Perfusion Ratio V/Q</u>
> V is higher at **base** of lung than at tip.
> Q is higher at **base** of lung than at tip.
> V/Q is higher at **tip** of lung than at base!
>
> (That's why tubercle bacilli are found at tips of lung
>   while pneumonia tends to develop at base of lungs.)

	OBSTRUCTIVE	RESTRICTIVE
VC	∅ or ↓	↓
FRC, RV	↑	↓
TLC	↑	↓

6.21.) BREATHING PATTERNS

Cheyne-Stokes	⩗	• **waxing and waning** • uremia • can be physiological at high altitude
Kussmaul	⩗	• **deep, fast inspirations** • compensation of metabolic acidosis (e.g. diabetic ketoacidosis)
Biot	⩗	• **apneic episodes** • brain tumors

Chronic lung disease (COPD):
→ central CO_2 receptors become less responsive.
→ peripheral O_2 receptors become "more important".
→ do not administer pure O_2 (patient may stop breathing!)

6.22.) RESPIRATORY CENTERS

EVIDENCE FROM EXPERIMENTAL TRANSSECTIONS:

IF YOU CUT:	→ CONSEQUENCE
above pons	normal respiration continues
above pons plus vagotomy	deeper inspirations (removal of afferent input from pulmonary sensory receptors)
mid pons	same effect as vagotomy
mid pons plus vagotomy	"apneusis" = arrested in inspiratory state [1]
below pons	irregular, fast and deep respiration (like gasping)
below medulla	all respirations seize

[1] *this finding suggests a "pneumotaxic center" located in the*
rostral pons which functions to limit the extent of inspirations.

6.23.) <u>RESPIRATORY QUOTIENT</u>
(= CO_2 release / O_2 uptake)

The respiratory quotient RQ is a simple indicator of the metabolic status of a patient and depends on diet:

	kcal / g	RQ
carbohydrates	4	1.0
proteins	4	0.8
fat	9	0.7

RQ < 0.7	• **hypoventilation** • diabetes • fasting
RQ > 1.0	• **hyperventilation**

6.24.) ACID-BASE

How to analyze acid-base abnormalities: (1.) Check the pH to determine whether it is an acidosis or alkalosis. (2.) Check whether the main abnormality (primary disturbance) is in PCO_2 levels (respiratory) or HCO_3^- (metabolic). In clinical practice it is rare to see a "pure" abnormality, most patients have at least some degree of compensation. (3.) If you want to be more sophisticated, you can determine from published charts whether the degree of compensation matches the degree of primary disturbance. If not, you have a combined disorder.

	pH	PRIMARY DISTURBANCE	COMPENSATORY RESPONSE	CLINICAL CONDITIONS
respiratory acidosis	< 7.35	PCO_2 ↑	HCO_3^- ↑	• sedation • sleep apnea • chest wall injuries • COPD
metabolic acidosis	< 7.35	HCO_3^- ↓	PCO_2 ↓	• ketoacidosis (diabetes) • lactacidosis (shock) • chronic diarrhea
respiratory alkalosis	> 7.45	PCO_2 ↓	HCO_3^- ↓	• anxiety • thyrotoxicosis • mountain climbing
metabolic alkalosis	> 7.45	HCO_3^- ↑	PCO_2 ↑	• loop diuretics (K^+ loss) • insulin (K^+ redistribution) • vomiting (H^+ loss)

<u>Salicylate intoxication</u>
Early: metabolic acidosis + respiratory alkalosis
Late: metabolic acidosis + respiratory acidosis

6.25.) <u>HEMOGLOBINS</u>

Hemoglobin is a protein consisting of 4 subunit chains, each containing one heme. Heme is an iron-containing porphyrin derivative that can bind one O_2 molecule (=oxyhemoglobin). Binding of O_2 is NOT a chemical oxidation of heme!

A) <u>PHYSIOLOGICAL</u>:

	HEMOGLOBIN	CHAINS
embryo	Gower 1	$\zeta_2\varepsilon_2$
fetus	HbF	$\alpha_2\gamma_2$
adult	HbA HbA$_2$ HbA$_{1C}$	$\alpha_2\beta_2$ (98%) $\alpha_2\delta_2$ (2%) glycosylated derivative

B) <u>PATHOLOGICAL</u>:

	HEMOGLOBIN	CHAINS
sickle cell anemia	HbS	$\alpha_2\beta^s_2$
α-thalassemia	HbH Hb Bart	β_4 γ_4
β-thalassemia	HbF HbA$_2$	$\alpha_2\delta_2$ $\alpha_2\gamma_2$

Sickle cell anemia is due to a point mutation of the β-chains. HbS forms polymers on deoxygenation, red cells loose their deformability and assume a sickled shape.

Hemoglobin is a major H^+ buffer of the blood. Deoxygenated hemoglobin is less acidic than oxygenated hemoglobin and therefore ideally suited to buffer the H^+ ions (coming from tissue CO_2) in the venous blood.

6.26.) <u>OXYGEN BINDING CURVE</u>

Sigmoidal relationship between PO_2 in blood and percent O_2 saturation of hemoglobin.

right shift	**= reduced binding of O_2** increased protons (low pH) increased CO_2 increased 2,3-DPG increased temperature
left shift	**= tighter binding of O_2** fetal hemoglobin [1] myoglobin [1]

[1] *for a given PO_2 fetal hemoglobin and myoglobin take up more O_2. As a result, O_2 is transferred from maternal Hb to fetal Hb and from Hb to myoglobin.*

	ARTERIAL	**VENOUS**
PO_2	95 mmHg	40 mmHg
O_2 saturation	97 %	70 %
PCO_2	40 mmHg	45 mm Hg
pH	7.4	7.37

6.27.) BLOOD PROTEINS

plasma = serum + clotting factors

Plasma is the fluid portion of blood. If whole blood is allowed to clot and the clot is removed, the remaining fluid is called serum. Plasma proteins can be separated by size by electrophoresis:

	FUNCTIONS	DECREASED IN:
prealbumin	• thyroxine, vitamin A	
albumin	• oncotic pressure • binds hormones, drugs	• malnutrition • liver failure • pregnancy
α1 globulin	• lipoproteins • α1 antitrypsin	• α1 deficiency
α2 globulin	• haptoglobin (carries hemoglobin dimers)	• Wilson's disease
β globulin	• transferrin (carries iron)	
γ globulin	• antibodies	• agammaglobulinemia

Low levels of blood protein (liver disease, nephrotic syndrome) result in edema due to loss of oncotic pressure.

334

6.28.) <u>CIRCULATION</u>

Perfusion of organs is under local control. Blood flow through the brain and kidneys is autoregulated, i.e. largely independent of blood pressure. Blood flow through skeletal muscle depends on metabolites: pH, lactate, ADP...

A) <u>PERFUSION</u>:

perfusion (rest) (in % of cardiac output)	kidney > brain, muscle > heart
perfusion (exercise) (in % of cardiac output)	muscle >> heart > brain > kidney
specific perfusion (rest) (in ml min^{-1} / g tissue)	kidney >> heart > brain > muscle

B) <u>PROPERTIES OF VESSELS</u>:

largest pressure	arteries
largest resistance	arterioles
largest cross-sectional area	capillaries
largest blood volume	veins

<u>Orthostasis (standing up)</u>
- systolic blood pressure unchanged
- diastolic blood pressure increased
- peripheral resistance increased
- heart rate increased

6.29.) <u>FETAL CIRCULATION</u>

Fetal circulation is characterized by a R → L shunt. Oxygenated blood from the placenta passes through the right atrium and open foramen ovale into the left atrium. Deoxygenated blood from the upper body passes through the right atrium, right ventricle, pulmonary artery to the ductus arteriosus and into the aorta.

foramen ovale	right atrium → left atrium
ductus arteriosus	pulmonary artery → aorta
ductus venosus	umbilical vein → vena cava inf.

> - Ductus arteriosus is kept open by prostaglandins.
> - Lung maturation is accelerated by glucocorticoids.

 Placenta receives 30-40% of fetal blood circulation.

 Head and upper extremities (<u>preductal</u>) receive O₂ rich blood. Lower extremities (<u>postductal</u>) receive mixed blood.

Head and upper extremities (<u>preductal</u>) receive O_2 rich blood. Lower extremities (<u>postductal</u>) receive mixed blood.

<u>HEMODYNAMICS AT BIRTH</u>
- Foramen ovale closes
  (left atrial pressure higher than right atrial pressure)
- Shunt reversal through ductus arteriosus L → R
  (aortic pressure higher than pulmonary artery pressure)
- Ductus arteriosus closes within a few months.

6.30.) RENAL TRANSPORT

The renal tubuli recover most of the filtered ions and small molecules and concentrate the urine to preserve water (anti-diuresis).

proximal tubule	• active resorption (glucose, amino acids etc.) • active secretion (organic acids, protons etc.) ➤ *carbonic anhydrase inhibitors act here*
Henle loop	• NaCl resorption • thick ascending portion is water impermeable! (generates osmotic gradient) ➤ *loop diuretics act here*
distal tubule	• K^+ secretion, H^+ secretion (in exchange for Na^+) ➤ *thiazide diuretics act here*
collecting duct	• water permeability under hormonal control • ADH increases permeability → water reabsorption ↑ → urine concentrated

RELATIONSHIP BETWEEN H⁺ AND K⁺

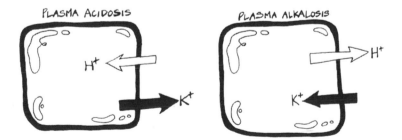

From Goldberg: *Clinical Physiology Made Ridiculously Simple*, MedMaster, 2007

EXCRETION OF H⁺ (proximal and distal tubule)

- **Titratable acids:** H^+ (<1%), uric acid (10%), phosphate (40%)
- **Non-titratable acids:** NH_4^+ (50%)

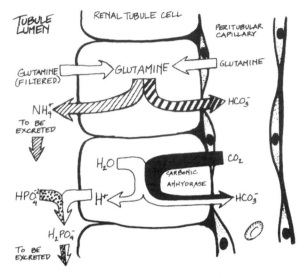

RECOVERY OF BICARBONATE (proximal tubule)

- 99.9% of filtered HCO_3^- is recovered.
- H^+ is secreted (in exchange for Na^+) and combines with tubular HCO_3^- forming H_2CO_3 which dissociates into H_2O and CO_2. CO_2 diffuses into the cell and is split back into H^+ for secretion and HCO_3^- which then is transported through the basolateral membrane (carrier mediated) into the peritubular space.

From Goldberg: *Clinical Physiology Made Ridiculously Simple*,
MedMaster, 2007

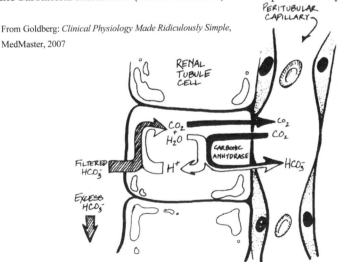

6.31.) <u>CLEARANCE</u>

Clearance is the amount of plasma (per minute) that gets <u>completely</u> "cleared". If a substance is completely removed from the plasma while passing through the kidneys, then its clearance equals renal plasma flow.

	NORMAL VALUE	CALCULATED FROM MEASUREMENT OF:
RBF (renal blood flow)	1,200 ml / min	PAH clearance and hematocrit
RPF (renal plasma flow)	600 ml / min	PAH clearance
GFR (glomerular filtration rate)	125 ml / min	inulin clearance or creatinine clearance
FF (filtration fraction)	20 %	GFR / RPF

	INTERPRETATION:
clearance > GFR	filtration + net secretion
clearance = GFR	filtration only (or secretion = resorption)
clearance < GFR	filtration + net resorption

- Contraction of afferent arteriole decreases GFR.
- Contraction of efferent arteriole increases GFR.

6.32.) <u>VOLUME REGULATION</u>

Plasma volume and osmolarity are closely linked: The most common cause of hyperosmolarity is dehydration (loss of water)!

	RECEPTORS	MECHANISM
osmoregulation	• hypothalamus	<u>hyperosmolarity results in:</u> • thirst • ADH release
volume regulation	• baroreceptors • macula densa	<u>blood volume loss results in:</u> • sympathetic activation • renin release from JGA

6.33.) <u>FLUID SHIFTS</u>

	ICV	ECV	CLINICAL EXAMPLES
hypotone dehydration	↑	↓	• diarrhea, vomiting[1]
isotone dehydration	Ø	↓	• blood loss
hypertone dehydration	↓	↓	• excessive sweating[2] • diabetes insipidus
hypotone hydration	↑	↑	• SIADH
isotone hydration	Ø	↑	• cardiac failure • nephrotic syndrome
hypertone hydration	↓	↑	• hyperaldosteronism

[1] *loss of NaCl large compared to loss of water*
[2] *loss of water large compared to electrolytes*

6.34.) <u>RENIN / ANGIOTENSIN</u>

The renin-angiotensin system is the most important regulator of blood volume. It is activated when renal blood flow decreases. In cardiac failure, it results in edema and congestion.

	PRODUCED BY:	**FEATURES:**
angiotensinogen	liver	$\alpha 2$ globulin
((renin))	kidney (JGA)	protease
angiotensin I		
((converting enzyme))	lung	protease
angiotensin II		vasoconstriction aldosterone release
aldosterone	zona glomerulosa	Na^+ reabsorption K^+ secretion
atrial natriuretic peptide (ANP)	heart: (high ECV → stretch of atria)	natriuresis
natriuretic factor (ouabain-like inhibitor of Na^+/K^+ pump)		unknown significance

Macula densa is a modified epithelium of distal tubule, juxtaglomerular.

Renin is released when: • blood pressure at JG cells is low.
                                • NaCl delivery to macula densa is low.

Patients with Bartter's syndrome:
• high renin, angiotensin and aldosterone, but normotensive!
  (down regulation of vascular angiotensin receptors???)

Patients with hypertension • respond to ACE inhibitors even when their
                                          renin levels are normal or low!

6.35.) JUXTAGLOMERULAR APPARATUS

The juxtaglomerular apparatus is named for its location next to the glomerulus. It is found between the afferent arteriole and the returning distal convoluted tubule of the same nephron. Three major cell types form this apparatus: (1.) **Macula densa cells** of the distal tubule which measure the sodium chloride concentration in the lumen. (2.) Specialized smooth muscle cells of the afferent arteriole (= **JG cells = granular cells**) which release renin. (3.) **Mesangial cells** of unknown function.

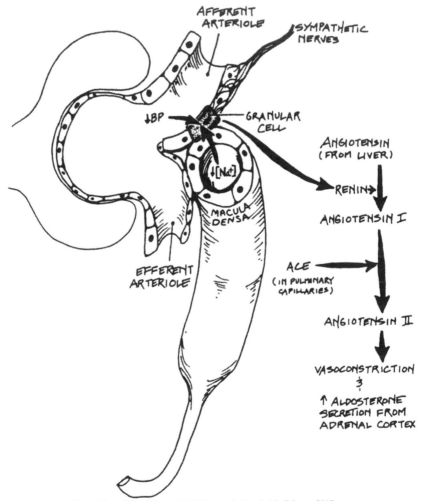

From Goldberg: *Clinical Physiology Made Ridiculously Simple*, MedMaster, 2007

6.36.) <u>INTESTINAL ABSORPTION</u>

The digestive and absorptive functions of the GI tract are essential for life. Resection of more than 50% of the small intestine leads to malabsorption and wasting. Reduced fat absorption results in vitamin deficiencies (A,D,E and K) and bulky, greasy, foul smelling stools.

carbohydrates	duodenum	jejunum	
amino acids	duodenum	jejunum	
iron	duodenum		
vit. B12			terminal ileum
bile salts			terminal ileum

<u>IRON</u>
- absorbed as Fe^{2+} (combine with anti-oxidants like vit. C)
- transported as transferrin
- stored as ferritin and hemosiderin

<u>DEFECTS OF AMINO ACID TRANSPORTERS</u>
- **Hartnup disease:** defect in neutral amino acid transporter
- **Cystinuria:** defect in basic amino acid transporter

6.37.) GI HORMONES

The gastrointestinal tract has its own nervous system and produces hormones which regulate its digestive functions:

	RELEASED BY:	RESULTS IN:
gastrin	• vagus nerve (ACh) • peptides, alcohol and alkaline pH in stomach	• HCl secretion • increased stomach motility • delayed stomach emptying
secretin	• acidic pH in duodenum	• HCO_3^- rich pancreatic secretion
CCK	• fat and peptides in duodenum	• enzyme rich pancreatic secretion • gallbladder contractions
GIP	• glucose, fat in duodenum	• stimulates insulin secretion
somatostatin	• acidic pH in stomach	• inhibits HCl secretion (stomach) • inhibits enzyme secretion (pancreas)

6.38.) STOMACH

	MAINLY SECRETES:
chief cells [1]	• pepsinogen
parietal cells [1]	• HCl • intrinsic factor
mucus cells [1,2]	• mucus
G cells [2]	• gastrin

[1] *fundus and corpus*   [2] *antrum*

344

6.39.) <u>PITUITARY FEEDBACK LOOPS</u>

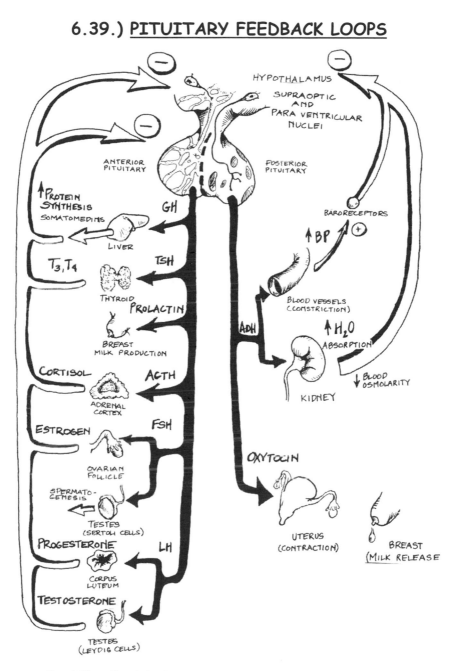

From Goldberg: *Clinical Physiology Made Ridiculously Simple*, MedMaster, 2007

6.40.) ADRENAL HORMONES

The adrenal cortex produces 2 vital hormones plus a small amount of androgens.
Overproduction or lack of these hormones results in important clinical syndromes:

	RELEASED BY:	SYNDROMES
aldosterone	• Angiotensin II • high K^+ ○ (ACTH)	**CONN** (=hyperaldosteronism) • K^+ depletion • hypertension ○ but not edematous ! ○ not hypernatremic ! • weakness, tetany **ADDISON** (hypoaldosteronism) • Na^+ loss (hypotension) • K^+ retention • H^+ retention (metabolic acidosis) • pigmentation
cortisol	• stress • ACTH	**CUSHING** (cortisol excess) • skin atrophy • muscle wasting • moon face • decreased glucose tolerance • poor wound healing • osteoporosis

*Most adrenalectomized patients could survive on mineralocorticoids
alone, but would face potentially fatal hypoglycemic episodes.*

Regulation Of Adrenal Hormone Release:

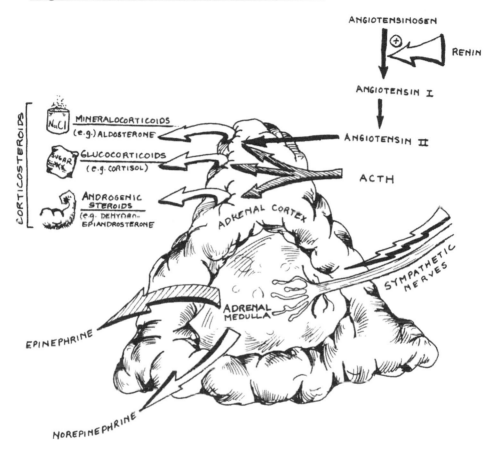

From Goldberg: *Clinical Physiology Made Ridiculously Simple*, MedMaster, 2007

Tumors of the adrenal medulla are called pheochromocytomas.

6.41.) INSULIN

Insulin is an anabolic hormone with a wide range of metabolic effects:

	LIVER	MUSCLE	FAT CELLS
carbohydrates	glycogen synthesis↑ gluconeogenesis↓	glucose transport↑ glycolysis↑ glycogen synthesis↑	glucose transport↑ glycerol synthesis↑
proteins		amino acid uptake↑ protein synthesis↑	
fat	lipogenesis↑		triglyceride synthesis↑ lipolysis↓

> ## THE INSULIN RECEPTOR
> α **subunit** binds insulin
> β **subunit** has tyrosine kinase activity:
> • phosphorylates itself (autophosphorylation)
> • phosphorylates many other proteins
> • activates ras → raf → MAP kinase cascade

6.42.) GONADOTROPE HORMONES

The gonads are under control of 2 hormones from the anterior pituitary gland. Estrogens suppress FSH (negative feedback). In infertile women, ovulation can sometimes be induced by giving an anti-estrogen.

	OVARIES	TESTES
FSH	follicle maturation	spermatogenesis
LH = ICSH	triggers ovulation luteinization of follicle	testosterone secretion (Leydig cells)

SOCIAL SCIENCES

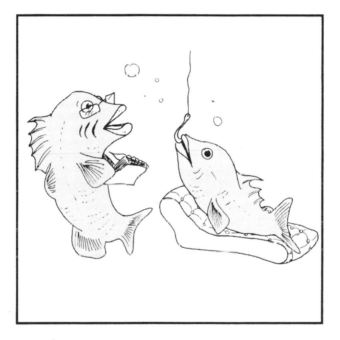

"And how long have you been feeling that people are after you?"

Part A : Psychology

7.1.) MOTOR DEVELOPMENT

The nervous system continues to mature after birth. Developmental milestones are important to assess in every infant:

chin up	1 month
chest up	2 month
knee push and "swim"	6 month
sits alone / stands with help	7 month
crawls on stomach	8 month
stands holding on furniture	10 month
walks when led	11 month
stands alone	14 month
walks alone	15 month

AT THE PLAYGROUND
- stranger anxiety: 0~1 years
- separation anxiety: 1~3 years
- parallel play: 2~3 years
- group play: 3~4 years

7.2.) PSYCHOLOGICAL DEVELOPMENT

years	Erikson	Freud	Piaget
0 - 1.5	trust vs. mistrust	oral (trust & dependence)	sensorimotor
1.5 - 3	autonomy vs. shame	anal (holding vs. letting out)	preoperational
3 - 6	initiative vs. guilt	phallic (Oedipus complex)	"
6 - 11	industry vs. inferiority	latency	concrete operational
11 - 20	identity vs. role confusion	genital (mature sexuality)	formal operational
20 - 25	intimacy vs. isolation		
25 - 50	generativity vs. stagnation		
50 - ?	integrity vs. despair		

MAJOR IDEAS:

Freud: Unconscious mental processes are the driving force motivating our behavior. Sexuality develops in stages, each stage focusing on a different body part.

Piaget: The thinking process develops in sequential stages, each stage qualitatively different from the others.

Erikson: The ego develops in stages over the entire lifetime. Each stage is characterized by a struggle that must be resolved before progressing to the next one.

7.3.) <u>IQ TESTS</u>

It is controversial whether intelligence is a single factor or composed of several independent factors and to what extend the IQ is determined genetically. There is a high concordance in monozygotic twins.

Deviation Tests	Tests of Mental Age
mean: 100 standard deviation: 15 normed for each age group	IQ = mental age / biological age
WAIS adults **WISC** children **WPPSI** preschool	**Stanford Binet** (for children and teenagers)

<u>Degrees of Mental Retardation</u>
In most cases the cause of mental retardation remains unknown.

IQ 55 - 70 (mild)	• mentally handicapped • educable
IQ 40 - 55 (moderate)	• trainable for personal hygiene
IQ 25 - 40 (severe)	• custodial
IQ < 25 (profound)	• custodial

7.4.) <u>CONDITIONING</u>

Behavior can be modified through experience (=learning). Major models of learning are the "classical conditioning" (Pavlov) and "operant conditioning" (Skinner).

CLASSICAL	OPERANT
<u>unconditioned:</u> **stimulus:** meat **response:** salivation	**operant:** behavior to be modified
<u>conditioned:</u> **stimulus:** bell **response:** salivation	positive reinforcer: candy negative reinforcer: shock **primary reward:** food, sex **secondary reward:** money, praise
• works on reflexive behavior (autonomic nervous system)	• works on autonomic nervous system or complex behavior
• reinforcement (unconditioned stimulus) occurs regardless of response	• reward / punishment depends on response
• partial reinforcement hastens extinction	• partial or variable reinforcement results in greater resistance to extinction (for example: gambling addiction…)

 Extinction*: Disappearance of learned behavior*

7.5.) DEFENSE MECHANISMS

Defense mechanisms are "normal", but there are mature ones (repression, rationalization) and immature ones (denial, temper tantrum). Symptoms or disease occur when defense mechanism break down or if the energy required to uphold the defenses becomes excessive.

- **Regression**
  Returning to immature ways of dealing with stress: crying, tantrums…
- **Repression**
  Blocking of unacceptable urges and feelings from awareness.
- **Denial**
  Blocking of unacceptable information or perceptions from awareness.
- **Rationalization**
  Substituting an acceptable motive for attitudes or behavior for an unacceptable motive.
- **Splitting**
  Maintaining a perception of others (or self) as all good or all bad.
- **Projection**
  "You are acting like a teenager, not I!"
- **Reaction formation**
  You want to 'kick his ass' but end up kissing it…
- **Isolation of affect**
  She talked about her baby's death calmly, without a sad expression.
- **Displacement**
  You are angry with your boss but shout at your kids instead.
- **Undoing**
  "Magic": knocking on wood etc.

> ### Transference
> Patient falls in love with therapist.
> ### Countertransference
> Therapist falls in love with patient.

 Always watch your countertransference!

7.6.) SLEEP STAGES

Sleep is important. Rats who are chronically deprived of sleep will die after few weeks. The role of REM sleep remains unclear. Suppression of REM sleep in volunteers appears to have no obvious ill effects.

	KEY FEATURES	EEG
awake		**beta:** > 12 / sec **alpha:** 8-12 / sec
stage 1		**theta:** 4-8 / sec
stage 2		low voltage sleep spindles
stages 3, 4	• night terrors • sleep walking • sleep talking o enuresis	**delta:** 1-4 / sec
REM	• rapid eye movements • paralysis of skeletal muscles (except eyes, finger, toes) • increased blood pressure and respiration • penis erection • dreams, nightmares	like awake state

---

Night terrors: extreme fright, no memory or dream

Narcolepsy: - patient suddenly falls asleep (REM at onset!)
      - cataplexy (sudden collapse because of loss of muscle tone)
      - hypnagogic hallucinations (just before falling asleep)
      - sleep paralysis (awake but unable to move or speak)

Sleep apnea: central: no respiratory effort
      obstructive: increased respiratory effort against
            airway obstruction

7.7.) <u>SUICIDE</u>

> <u>Risk factors:</u>   - has specific plan (always ask!)
>   - lack of social support
>   - recovery phase of depression
>   - physicians, dentists

- success-rate: ~10%
- after failed attempts: 30% will try again
- 80% have given warning

○ **women:** more overall attempts than men
○ **men:** more "successful" suicides than women
○ more common in **elderly**
○ more common in **single** than in married people
○ more common in **divorced** than in single people

<u>LEADING CAUSES OF DEATH</u>:

White teenagers: motor vehicle accidents > suicides > homicides
Black teenagers: homicides > motor vehicle accidents > suicides

7.8.) <u>STAGES OF DYING</u>
Elisabeth Kübler-Ross

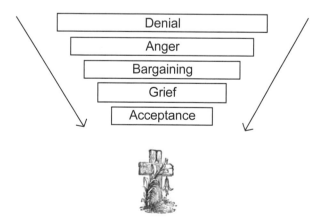

Part B :
Psychopathology

7.9.) NEUROTRANSMTTERS

Most major psychiatric diseases are associated with abnormal levels of neuro-transmitters. Whether these changes are the actual cause of psychiatric disease remains controversial.

	NEUROTRANSMITTER LEVELS:
schizophrenia	• dopamine ↑
depression	• norepinephrine ↓ • serotonin ↓ • dopamine ↓
Alzheimer's disease	• acetylcholine ↓ (nucleus of Meynert)
anxiety	• GABA ↓

Benzodiazepines and barbiturates act on GABA receptors:
→ open Cl⁻ channels
→ hyperpolarization of nerve cell
→ decreased neuronal firing

7.10.) GRIEF & DEPRESSION

Grief is a normal reaction caused by loss and does not reach the level of clinical depression.

GRIEF	MAJOR DEPRESSION
• initial: shock/denial • illusions / hallucinations may occur • low risk of suicide	• feeling of hopelessness • feeling of worthlessness • high risk of suicide

Abnormal grief reaction:
- continued thoughts about guilt and death
- marked psychomotor retardation
- marked functional impairment
- lasts < 2 months (if longer, a diagnosis of
   major depression is likely)

7.11.) DELIRIUM & DEMENTIA

Delirium is often caused by toxins, metabolites or infections.
Dementia most commonly is due to Alzheimer's or cerebrovascular disease.

DELIRIUM	DEMENTIA
• impaired consciousness (agitation or stupor)	• unimpaired consciousness
• develops quickly, fluctuating	• slow, progressive
• usually reversible	• irreversible

7.12.) <u>PERSONALITY DISORDERS</u>

Inflexible, rigid behavioral pattern that causes social impairment. Begins during adolescence and patients are usually NOT distressed and do NOT seek help.

A) <u>ECCENTRIC</u>:

paranoid	• patient projects his fears onto others • may blame physician or others for disease
schizoid	• anxious, withdrawn • doesn't want close relationships
schizotypal	• odd ideas, paranoia, magical thinking • premorbid personality type of schizophrenics

B) <u>EMOTIONAL, DRAMATIC</u>:

histrionic	• dramatic, emotional • may display inappropriate sexual behavior
narcissistic	• feels better than others • perfect self-image is threatened by disease
borderline	• severe disorder with features of psychoses • intense, unstable relationships • self-damaging, suicidal

C) <u>FEARFUL, ANXIOUS</u>:

dependent	• afraid of being helpless • need to be cared for
compulsive	• fear of loss of control • tries to control physician
avoidant	• hypersensitive to rejection or failure • fear starting relationships • strong desire for affection

7.13.) <u>ANXIETY DISORDERS</u>

Fear is an emotional and physiological response to a real threat; anxiety is a similar response without a clear external threat. Patients with anxiety disorders are distressed and know that their symptoms are irrational.

phobia	• persistent excessive fear of <u>specific</u> objects or situations • patient knows that his fear his unrealistic
Agoraphobia [1]	• history of panic attacks • patient <u>avoids</u> places were panic attacks might occur (especially public places)
obsessive-compulsive	• **obsessions:** recurrent thoughts • **compulsions:** repetitive behavior
posttraumatic stress disorder	• traumatic event in history • may occur ANY time after event • persists for > 1 month
generalized anxiety disorder	• excessive anxiety and worries • restlessness, muscle tension, irritability

[1] *strictly speaking, this is NOT a phobia!*

7.14.) SOMATOFORM DISORDERS

Physical symptoms without organic pathology, causing significant
distress or functional impairment.

somatization
(Briquet's syndrome)
	• sickly for most of life
	• involves <u>many organ systems</u>:
	  - gastrointestinal
	  - cardiopulmonary
	  - reproductive
	  - pain
	
	• diagnosis requires at least 12 symptoms
	      PLUS
	• history of several years.

conversion disorder (hysterical neurosis)	• "<u>pseudo-neurological</u>" (blindness, paresthesia, paralysis) • symptoms begin and end suddenly • often misdiagnosed as "malingering"
hypochondriasis	• <u>unrealistic interpretation</u> of body signs • belief to have serious disease that goes unrecognized by family and physicians

7.15.) <u>SCHIZOPHRENIA</u>

Psychotic illness with disorganized thinking, speech and behavior. 1% risk among general population, 15% for persons who have a 1st degree relative with schizophrenia. Leads to progressive mental deterioration ("dementia praecox")

positive symptoms:	• delusions • hallucinations (often auditory)
negative symptoms:	• flat affect • avolition
"four A's":	• affect inappropriate • ambivalence • associative thinking (alogical) • autism

7.16.) <u>MAJOR DEPRESSION</u>

Severe mood disorder that is qualitatively different from normal grief or sadness. Abnormalities in biorhythms and sleep pattern are very common in these patients.

major depression	• depressed mood • feeling of worthlessness • weight loss! • early morning insomnia!
bipolar type-1	• at least <u>one manic</u> episode in patient's history
bipolar type-2	• at least <u>one major depressive</u> episode PLUS at least <u>one hypomanic or manic</u> episode

You should NOT make diagnosis of major depression within two months after bereavement (loss of a loved-one), even if the "classical" symptoms are present!

7.17.) EPILEPSY

Brief attacks of altered consciousness, motor activity and sensation caused by excessive discharge of cerebral neurons. Tonic-clonic seizures are the most common (90%).

grand mal	• tonic, then clonic • loss of consciousness • incontinence EEG : high voltage spikes
petit mal	• absence seizure ("blank spell") • no loss of muscle tone EEG : 3/sec spikes and domes
narcolepsy	• loss of muscle tone • REM onset sleep
psychomotor	• non-goal directed activity (lip smacking, walking...) EEG : spikes in temporal lobes
Jacksonian	• spreading muscle group activity (e.g. fingers → forearm → shoulder) EEG : focus around antral sulcus

7.18.) DRUG ABUSE

Abuse: Recurrent use of drugs resulting in (1.) social failures at home,
school or work, (2.) legal problems (3.) hazardous situations.
Dependence: Tolerance - needs larger doses to achieve effect
- severe withdrawal symptoms

	INTOXICATION	WITHDRAWAL
alcohol	• euphoria • disorientation • unsteady gait	• nausea • tremor, seizures • delusions, hallucinations • delirium tremens
barbiturates	• sedation	• can be severe! • delirium • epilepsy • coma, death
benzodiazepines	• antianxiety • sedation	• anxiety • irritability • insomnia
amphetamines, cocaine	• arousal • euphoria	• fatigue • dysphoria
opioids	• euphoria • apathy	• nausea, vomiting • sweating, fever • muscle ache
LSD	• hallucinations • anxiety • paranoid ideas	none

Blood alcohol: > 0.1% → intoxication
> 0.2% → fall asleep, anesthesia
> 0.4% → inhibition of respiration, death

 Typical metabolic rate is 10~20 mg/dL (0.01~0.02%) per hour.

7.19.) <u>CHILD ABUSE</u>

More than 1 million reported cases per year in the US! Abuse can be physical, emotional or sexual. Neglect is the failure to meet the child's physical or medical needs.

PHYSICAL	SEXUAL
• infants, younger children	• preadolescent, adolescents
• abuser often female	• abuser usually male
	• abuser usually known to victim
RISK FACTORS:	**RISK FACTORS:**
- prematurity, low birth weight	- drug abuse
- drug abuse	- single-parent home
- parents abused as children [1]	
- poverty	

[1] *unable to give what they never received...*

PERHAPS ACCIDENTAL	MORE LIKELY INTENTIONAL
• splash marks	• clearly demarcated areas, no splash
• injuries to front	• injuries to back
• foot soles spared	• foot soles involved
	• history of multiple injuries
	• retinal hemorrhage ("shaken baby")

 Report to Social Department, but do not play "detective"!

365

Part C : Statistics

The USMLE does not require you to do complicated statistical calculations, but you need to know the definitions and when to apply which test.

7.20.) DEFINITIONS

Standard deviation: ±1s includes 68%, ±2s includes 95%, ±3s includes 99%

Mean: average value
Median: half the values are higher, half the values are lower than this
Mode: most common value
(In a perfectly symmetrical distribution, mean, median and mode are the same!)

Relative risk: (incidence with risk factor) / (incidence without risk factor)
Attributable risk: (incidence with risk factor) - (incidence without risk factor)

Chi square test. Analysis of categorical data distribution.
- *Example: Two groups of patients with chronic arthritis are given either drug or placebo. Condition after treatment will be rated "improved", "same", or "worsened".*

Paired Student's t-test. Each patient serves as its own control.
- *Example: A group of patients with hypertension is treated first with placebo then with drug (or vice versa) in a "cross-over" design.*

Correlation coefficient. Test of degree of association between two variables.
- *Example: BP and triglyceride levels are measured in a cross-sectional study of patients.*

Analysis of variance. Determine how several independent variables affect one dependent variable (similar to t-test, but more variables).
- *Example: Effect of blood pressure, cholesterol, triglycerides and patient's income on incidence of myocardial infarction.*

Analysis of covariance. Determine how several independent variables affect one dependent variable and controlling for other variables.
- *Example: Assessment of effect of drug versus placebo in two groups of patients taking pretreatment blood pressure into account.*

7.21.) <u>SENSITIVITY</u>

Sensitivity = probability that a sick patient (A ı C) will have a positive test result (A).

	patient is sick	patient is healthy
test result is positive	A	B
test result is negative	C	D

Sensitivity: divide A by (A+C)

C = "False negative"

> ➤ Tests with high sensitivity are used for screening.
> ➤ Tests with high sensitivity are used to "rule out" diagnosis.

"*A test has a sensitivity of 90%*" means that 10% of patients with the disease go undetected (false negative).

7.22.) <u>SPECIFICITY</u>

Specificity = probability that a healthy patient (B+D) will have a
negative test result (D).

	patient is sick	patient is healthy
test result is positive	A	B
test result is negative	C	D

Specificity: divide D by (B+D)

B = "False positive"

> ➤ Tests with high specificity are used to confirm diagnosis.

 "A test has a specificity of 80%" means that 20% of people
without disease get a false positive test result.

 Sensitivity and specificity are <u>independent</u> of disease
prevalence!

7.23.) <u>POSITIVE PREDICTIVE VALUE</u>

PPV = probability that a patient with a positive test result (A+B)
is indeed sick (A).

	patient is sick	patient is healthy
test result is positive	A	B
test result is negative	C	D

Positive predictive value: divide A by (A+B)

> ➤ The predictive value depends not only on the test's properties
>   but also on disease prevalence.
> ➤ PPV is higher in populations with high prevalence!

*If you had screened inhabitants of Siberia in 1985 for HIV
antibodies, all positive results would have been false positive and
the PPV would have been 0.*

*Screening an asymptomatic, low-risk population will result in
many false positives. The expense for follow-up of false positive
results (plus the alarm you cause the patient) needs to be weighed
against the benefits of early disease detection.*

7.24.) <u>NEGATIVE PREDICTIVE VALUE</u>

NPV = probability that a patient with a negative test result (C+D) is indeed healthy (D).

	patient is sick	patient is healthy
test result is positive	A	B
test result is negative	C	D

Negative predictive value: divide D by (C+D)

> ➤ The predictive value depends not only on the test's properties but also on disease prevalence.
> ➤ NPV is higher in populations with low prevalence!

7.25.) <u>CANCER STATISTICS (USA)</u>

The most common cancer is basal cell carcinoma of the skin. Because of its low metastatic potential (<0.01%) it is not considered on "cancer statistics".

A.) <u>Incidence</u>
= number of <u>new</u> people that develop disease
in one year per 100,000 population

MALE	FEMALE
1. prostate (41%)	1. breast (31%)
2. lung (13%)	2. lung (13%)
3. colorectal (9%)	3. colorectal (11%)

B.) <u>Mortality</u>
= number of people who die of disease
in one year per 100,000 population

MALE	FEMALE
1. lung (32%)	1. lung (25%)
2. prostate (14%)	2. breast (17%)
3. colorectal (9%)	3. colorectal (10%)

C.) <u>Prevalence</u>
= number of people who have disease
at a given date (or time interval) per 100,000 population

• depends on both incidence and duration of disease

7.26.) <u>RANDOMIZED CLINICAL TRIAL</u>

"State of the Art" test to evaluate new drugs.

design	• researcher conducts interventions
study group	• patients are selected and assigned randomly to intervention or control groups
observation	• patients are assessed before and after intervention or control procedure

Null hypothesis:	assumes that there is no significant difference between new drug and control treatment
Type I error:	null hypothesis is rejected although it is true *(i.e. to claim that drug is effective when it is not)*
Type II error:	null hypothesis is not rejected even though it is false *(i.e. to claim that drug is not effective when it really is)*
P value:	probability of a type I error

 P=0.05 means that there is a 5% probability that the observed difference between new drug and control treatment was due to chance. The lower the P value the better.

 The larger the number of patients in the study, the lower P tends to be.

7.27.) <u>OBSERVATIONAL COHORT</u>
(prospective)

Used to estimate incidence of disease in groups with different risk factors.

design	• researcher observes natural events over time • no intervention, but requires lots of time and effort
study group	• two patient groups defined by presence/absence of risk factors are compared
observation	• patients are assessed repeatedly during course of study for incidence of disease

Validity: does the test measure what it is supposed to measure?
Reliability: how well can the test results be reproduced?

Framingham Heart Study
- sample population of Framingham, Massachusetts
- assesses risk factors for cardiovascular disease
- began in 1950, still ongoing today!

7.28.) CASE CONTROL STUDY

(retrospective)

Used to identify risk factors.

design	• researcher determines presence of risk factors retrospectively
study group	• two patient groups defined by presence/absence of disease are compared
observation	• patients are assessed for presence of disease at begin of study, then questioned for risk factors

7.29.) CROSS SECTIONAL SURVEY

(convenient, common study)

Used to determine correlations between two or more variables.

design	• researcher records presence of variables • can be done on existing data base
study group	• single patient group for which association between variables is sought
observation	• data are obtained on all variables of interest at the same point of time

Correlation coefficient: +1 perfect correlation
0 no correlation between variables
-1 perfect negative correlation

7.30.) LEGAL ISSUES

- **Competent patients** may refuse medical treatment, even if death will result.

- **Involuntary treatment** requires   a) patient is mentally ill
                                                      PLUS
                                     b) danger to self or others

- **Confidentiality:** May be breached if significant risk to others exists:
                 (HIV positive prostitute, patient threatens to kill, child abuse)

- **Living will:** Directions for future care (when unable to make decisions)
- **Durable power of attorney:** designate a legal representative to make decisions

---

- **Minors:** Parents must give consent
No consent necessary if: - emergency
                                - pregnancy
                                - treatment of sexually transmitted diseases

- Some States require parental consent for abortion, others do not.

- Self-supporting minors are considered adults → parental consent is not required.

- **Medicare:** Care for the elderly (>65 years, part of "Social Security")
- **Medicaid:** Aid for the poor (on Welfare)

- **HMOs:** - prepaid insurance plan
                - physicians are paid fixed salary to take care of group of people

ABBREVIATIONS

a/w	associated with
AA	amyloid associated protein
Ab	antibodies
ACh	acetylcholine
ADHD	attention deficit hyperactivity disorder
AFP	alpha fetoprotein
AL	amyloid light chains
ALA	aminolevulinic acid
ANA	antinuclear antibodies
AP	action potential
aPTT	partial thromboplastin time
ASD	atrial septal defect
ARDS	acute respiratory distress syndrome
BP	blood pressure
CA	carcinoma
CEA	carcinoembryonic antigen
CoA	coenzyme A
COPD	chronic obstructive pulmonary disease
CSF	cerebrospinal fluid
CNS	central nervous system
DES	diethylstilbestrol
DIC	disseminated intravascular coagulation
DOC	drug of choice
ds	double stranded
DX	differential diagnosis
EBV	Epstein-Barr virus
ECV	extracellular volume
EEE	eastern equine encephalitis
G6PD	glucose-6-phosphate dehydrogenase
GABA	gamma-aminobutyrate
GBM	glomerular basement membrane
GH	growth hormone
GI	gastrointestinal
GN	glomerulonephritis
HCG	human chorionic gonadotropin
IDDM	insulin dependent diabetes mellitus
JGA	juxtaglomerular apparatus
LMN	lower motor neuron
LSD	lysergic acid diethylamide
MAC	minimal alveolar concentration
MAO	monoamine oxidase
MHC	major histocompatibility complex
MI	myocardial infarction
MIF	Müllerian inhibiting factor
MLC	myosin light chain
MODY	maturity onset diabetes of the young
MS	multiple sclerosis
NGU	non-gonorrheal urethritis
NIDDM	non insulin dependent diabetes mellitus
NSAID	nonsteroidal antiinflammatory drug
PAH	p-aminohippurate
PAS	periodic acid Schiff reagent
PCP	phencyclidine
PDA	patent ductus arteriosus
PDE	phosphodiesterase
PG	prostaglandin
PMN	polymorph nuclear leukocyte
PT	prothrombin time
RBC	red blood cells
RSV	respiratory syncytial virus
SLE	systemic lupus erythematosus
ss	single stranded
SSPE	subacute sclerosing panencephalitis
TCA	tricyclic antidepressants
THC	tetrahydrocannabinol
TIA	transient ischemic attack
TLC	total lung capacity
TPA	tissue plasminogen activator
TRAP	tartrate resistant alkaline phosphatase
TT	thrombin time
TX	treatment
UMN	upper motor neuron
UTI	urinary tract infection
VD	venereal disease
VDRL	Venereal Disease Research Laboratory
VSD	ventricular septal defect
VZV	varicella zoster virus
WEE	western equine encephalitis

INDEX

Anemia, 1.21, **1.28**
Anesthetics, **3.50**
Aneurysms, **1.38**
Angelman syndrome, 1.19
Angina, 1.41, 3.24
Angiotensin, **6.34**
Angiotensin antagonists, **3.21**
Ankle, **5.20**
Ankle jerk reflex, 5.42
Ankylosing spondylitis, 1.20
Anomers, 4.7
Antacids, 3.35
Anthrax, 2.12, 3.6
Antianginal drugs, **3.24**
Antiarrhythmic drugs, **3.28**
Antibiotics, **3.5**
Anticoagulants, **3.26**
Antidepressants, **3.44**
Antidotes, **3.4**
Antiemetic drugs, **3.54**
Antiepileptic drugs, **3.53**
Anti-folates, 3.14
Antifungal drugs, **3.10**
Antigenic drift, 2.25
Antigenic shift, 2.25
Antihistamines, **3.49**
Antihypertensive drugs, **3.20**
Antiprotozoal drugs, **3.11**
Antitoxin, 3.4
Antiviral drugs, **3.9**
Anxiety disorders, **7.13**
Anxiolytic drugs, **3.47**
Aortic regurgitation, 1.39
Aortic stenosis, 1.39
Aphasias, 5.27
Aplastic anemia, 1.28
Appendicitis, 5.24
Arachidonic acid, 4.15
ARBO viruses, **2.26**
ARDS, 1.48
Arsenic, 1.93
Arteriosclerosis, **1.36**
Arteritis, **1.37**
Arthritis, **1.75**
Arthus reaction, 1.8
Asbestos, 1.93

Ascaris, 2.39
Aschoff body, 1.46
Aseptic necrosis, 1.76
Aspergillosis, 2.32
Aspirin, 3.17, 3.25, 6.24
Astemizole, 3.49
Asthma, 1.47, **3.30**
Astrocytoma, 1.80
Atenolol, 3.36
Atherosclerosis, 1.36
Atonic bladder, 3.38
ATP equivalents, 4.26
Atrial natriuretic peptide, 6.34
Atrial septal defect, 1.40
Atropine, 3.39
Atypical pneumonia, 1.49, 3.6
Auditory meatus, 5.7
Autoantibodies, **1.6**
Automatic bladder, 3.38
Autonomic nervous system, **6.11**
Autosomal dominant diseases, **1.15**
Autosomal recessive diseases, **1.14**
Azathioprine, 3.14
AZT, 3.9, 3.12, 4.42

B
Bacilli, **2.11**
Bacillus anthracis, 2.12
Bactericidal, 3.5
Bacteriostatic, 3.5
Bacteroides fragilis, 2.15
Barbiturates, 3.48, 7.9, 7.18
Basal cell carcinoma, 1.91
Basal ganglia, **5.34**
Basilar skull fractures, 5.7
Basophil stippling, 1.29
Becker's dystrophy, 1.16, 1.79
Bence-Jones protein, 1.34
Benzene, 1.93
Benzodiazepines, 3.4, 3.47, 7.9, 7.18
Benztropine, 3.51
Berger's disease, 1.51
Berry aneurysms, 1.15
Beta-agonists, 3.29, 3.36
Beta-blockers, 3.20, 3.36
Beta-lactamase, 3.7

Beta-receptors, 6.13
Bethanechol, 3.38
Bicarbonate, 6.1, 6.30
Bile acids, **4.16**
Biot respiration, 6.21
Biperiden, 3.51
Bipolar disorder, 7.16
Bismuth, 3.35
Bladder, urinary, 3.38
Blastomycosis, 2.32
Bleeding disorders, **1.26**
Bleomycin, 3.14, 3.16
Blood alcohol, 7.18
Blood pressure, 6.11
Blood proteins, **6.27**
Bone diseases, **1.76**
Bone marrow suppression, 3.3
Bone tumors, **1.78**
Borderline personality, 7.12
Bordetella, 2.18
Bornholm disease, 2.26
Borrelia burgdorferi, 2.20
Botulinum toxin, 2.5
Botulism, 2.13
Bovine spongiform encephalopathy, 2.28
Bowel infarction, 5.22
Bowen's disease, 1.91
Brachial plexus, **5.13, 5.14, 5.15**
Brain tumors, **1.80**
Brainstem syndromes, **5.36 - 5.39**
Branchial arches, **5.3**
BRCA, 1.59
Breast diseases, **1.59**
Breathing patterns, **6.21**
Bretylium, 3.28
Briquet's syndrome, 7.14
Broca, 5.26
Bromocriptine, 3.22, 3.51
Bronchiectasis, 1.47
Bronchitis, 1.47, 2.7
Bronchopneumonia, 1.49
Brucella, 2.16
Bruton's agammaglobulinemia, 1.16, 1.25
Burkitt lymphoma, 1.9, 1.33, 2.24
Buspirone, 3.47

Butyrophenone, 3.52

C
C. donovani, 1.54
Cadmium, 1.93
Caffeine, 3.46
Calcium channel blockers, 3.20
Calories, 4.26
cAMP, 6.4
Campylobacter jejuni, 2.15, 3.6
Cancer statistics, **7.25**
Candida, 1.54, 2.32, 3.6, 3.10, 3.12
Captopril, 3.21
Carbachol, 3.38
Carbamazepine, 3.53
Carbenicillin, 3.7
Carbidopa, 3.51
Carbinoxamine, 3.49
Carbon monoxide, 3.4
Carbonic anhydrase inhibitors, 3.23
Carcinoid, 1.50
Cardiac cycle, **6.19**
Cardiac index, 6.1
Cardiac output, 6.1
Cardiolipin, 4.18
Carpal tunnel syndrome, 5.15
Cartilage, **1.77**
Case control studies, **7.28**
Castor oil, 3.55
Cat bites, 2.16
Catabolic, 4.41
Catalase, 2.8
Cataplexy, 7.6
Cauda equina lesion, 5.39
CCK, 6.37
CEA, 1.11
Cefamandole, 3.8
Cefazolin, 3.8
Cefotaxime, 3.8
Cefoxitin, 3.8
Ceftriaxone, 3.8
Celiac sprue, 1.6, 1.66
Celiac trunk, 5.23
Cell capsule, 2.4
Cell walls, **2.4**
Cellulose, 4.9

382

Familial polyposis, 1.15, 1.64
Famotidine, 3.35
Fanconi anemia, 1.28
Farsightedness, 6.7
Fasting, 4.24
Fatty acids, **4.15**
Febrile seizures, 3.53
Felty's syndrome, 1.30, 1.75
Femur neck fractures, 5.18
Fentanyl, 3.43
Fetal alcohol syndrome, 1.40
Fetal circulation, **6.29**
Fetal hydantoin syndrome, 1.40
Fetal remnants, **5.2**
Fever, 1.3
Fibers, 3.55
Fibroadenoma, 1.59
Fibrocystic change, 1.59
Fibrosis of lung, 1.48
Filtration fraction, 6.31
Flecainide, 3.28
Flora, normal, **2.3**
Flukes, **2.37**
Fluorouracil, 3.14, 4.44
Fluoxetine, 3.44
Fluphenazine, 3.52
Food poisoning, 1.21
Foot drop, 5.20
Foramen magnum, 5.7
Foramen ovale, 5.7, 6.29
Foramen rotundum, 5.7
Foramen spinosum, 5.7
Fragile X, 1.16
Framingham heart study, 7.27
Francisella, 2.16
Frank Starling mechanism, 6.14
Freud, 7.2
Friedreich's ataxia, 1.81
Fructose intolerance, 4.10, 4.11
Fructosuria, 4.10
FSH, 6.42
Fungal diseases, **2.32**, 3.10
Fungi, **2.31**
Furanose, 4.7
Furosemide, 3.23

G

G proteins, **6.4**
G6PD deficiency, 1.16, 1.27, 3.3
Galactosemia, 4.10, 4.11
Gallbladder carcinoma, **1.68**
Ganciclovir, 3.9
Gardner's syndrome, 1.64
Gastric ulcer, 3.6
Gastrin, 6.37
Gastritis, **1.62**
Gastroenteritis, **1.63**
Gastrointestinal hormones, **6.37**
Gaucher's disease, 4.20
Gene expression, **4.45**
Genetics of disease, **1.13**
Genital herpes, 1.54
Germ cell tumors, 1.55
Germ layers, **5.1**
German measles, 2.25
Gestational diabetes, 1.89
Ghon complex, 2.18
Giant cell arteritis, 1.37
Giardia lamblia, 2.35
Giemsa, 2.2
Gilbert's syndrome, 1.69
GIP, 6.37
Glioblastoma, 1.80
Glipizide, 3.32
Globulin, 6.27
Glomerular filtration rate, 6.31
Glomerulonephritis, **1.51**
Glomerulonephritis, **1.52**
Glossitis, 1.60
Glucagon, 4.41
Glucogenic, 4.3
Glucokinase, **4.8**
Glyburide, 3.32
Glycerophosphate shuttle, 4.26
Glycogen, 4.9
Glycogen storage diseases, 1.14, **4.12**
Glycolipids, **4.19**
Glycosaminoglycans, **4.14**
Glycosides, 3.29
Gold, 3.17

Golgi tendon organ, 6.16
Gonadotrope hormones, **6.42**
Gonococcus, 2.10
Gonorrhea, 3.6
Goodpasture syndrome, 1.6, 1.48, 1.51
Gout, **3.18**
Gower's sign, 1.79
gp120, 2.30
gp41, 2.30
Gram stain, 2.1
Gram-negative bacilli, **2.16**, **2.17**
Gram-positive bacilli, **2.12**
Grand mal, 3.53, 7.17
Granuloma inguinale, 1.54
Granulosa cells, **4.35**
Graves' disease, 1.6, 1.86
Grief, **7.10**
Griseofulvin, 3.10
Group play, 7.1
Growth hormone, 4.41
Guanethidine, 3.36
Guanylyl cyclase, 6.4
Guillain-Barré syndrome, 1.82, 5.39

H
H⁺, kidneys, 6.30
Hairy cell leukemia, 1.32
Hallucinogens, **3.42**
Haloperidol, 3.52
Halothane, 1.72, 3.50
Hamstrings, 5.19
Hand-foot-mouth disease, 2.25
Hantavirus, 2.26
Hartnup disease, 4.5
Hashimoto's thyroiditis, 1.6, 1.86
Heart beat, **6.14**
Heart failure, **1.43**
Heart muscle, **6.18**
Heart sounds, **1.39**
Heberden's nodes, 1.75
Heinz bodies, 1.29
Helicase, 4.47
Helicobacter pylori, 1.62, 2.15, 3.35
Hemangioblastoma, 1.80
Hemangioma, 1.92
Hematopoiesis, 1.4

Hemianopsia, 5.28
Hemochromatosis, 1.14, 1.20, 1.73, 1.89
Hemoglobin, **6.25**
Hemolytic anemias, **1.27**
Hemophilia, 1.16, 1.26
Hemophilus, 2.17
Hemophilus ducreyi, 1.54
Hemorrhage, intracranial, **5.30**
Henderson-Hasselbalch equation, 6.1
Henle loop, 6.30
Hepadnavirus, 2.23
Heparin, 3.4, 3.26
Hepatitis, **1.70**
Hepatitis serology, **1.71**
Hepatotoxicity, 3.3
Herpangina, 2.25
Herpes, 3.12
Herpes viruses, **2.24**
Heterophil negative mononucleosis, 2.24
Hexokinase, **4.8**
Hexoses, 4.7
Higher bacteria, **2.19**
Hip, **5.18**
Histoplasmosis, 2.32
Histrionic personality, 7.12
HIV, **2.30**, 3.12
HLA, **1.20**
HMOs, 7.30
Hodgkin's disease, 1.33, 3.16
Homocystinuria, 4.5, 4.6
Horner's syndrome, 5.8
Howell-Jolly bodies, 1.29
HPV, 1.54
HSV, 1.54, 2.24
Humerus fracture, 5.15
Hunter syndrome, 4.14
Huntington's disease, 1.15, 1.81, 5.34
Hurler syndrome, 4.14
Hutchinson's teeth, 1.40
Hydatidiform mole, 1.58
Hydrochlorothiazide, 3.23
Hydroxysteroids, 4.30
Hyperlipidemia, **3.33**, **3.34**
Hypermetropia, 6.7
Hypersensitivity, **1.8**
Hypersensitivity arteritis, 1.37

Hypersensitivity pneumonitis, 1.48
Hypertension, 1.21
Hypnagogic hallucinations, 7.6
Hypnotic drugs, **3.48**
Hypochondriasis, 7.14
Hypoglossal canal, 5.7
Hypoglossal nerve, 5.9
Hypoglycemic reaction, 3.31
Hysterical neurosis, 7.14
Ibuprofen, 3.17

I
ICSH, 6.42
IDDM, 1.20, 1.89
Idoxuridine, 3.9
IgA deficiency, 1.25
Immunodeficiencies, **1.25**
Impetigo, 1.92
Incidence, 7.25
India ink, 2.2
Indomethacin, 3.17
Inducers, 4.45
Infectious mononucleosis, 2.24
Inflammation, **1.3**
Inflammatory bowel disease, **1.65**
Influenza, 2.25
Inotropic drugs, **3.29**
Insulin, **3.31**, 4.41, **6.41**
Insulin receptor, 6.41
Interferon, 3.9
Internal carotid artery, 5.29
Intestinal absorption, **6.36**
Ion channels, **6.2**
IP3, 6.4
IQ tests, **7.3**
Iron, 3.4, 6.36
Iron deficiency anemia, 1.28
Ischemic heart disease, **1.41**
Isoflurane, 3.50
Isolation of affect, 7.5
Isometric contraction, 6.17
Isoniazid, 1.72
Isoproterenol, 3.36
Isosorbide dinitrate, 3.24
Isotonic contraction, 6.17

Isotretinoin, 1.40
ITP, 1.26
Itraconazole, 3.10

J
Jacksonian seizures, 7.17
Janeway lesions, 1.44
Jaundice, **1.69**
Jugular foramen, 5.7
Juvenile rheumatoid arthritis, 1.20

K
Kala-Azar, 2.34
Kaposi sarcoma, 2.24
Kartagener's, 1.47
Kawasaki, 1.37
Keratoacanthoma, 1.91
Ketamine, 3.50
Ketoconazole, 3.10
Ketogenic, 4.3
Ketosteroids, 4.30
Key enzymes, **4.27, 4.28, 4.29**
Klebsiella, 2.15
Knee, **5.19**
Knee jerk reflex, 5.42, 6.16
Koplik's spots, 1.60
Krabbe's disease, 4.20
Kübler-Ross, 7.8
Kuru, 2.28
Kussmaul respiration, 6.21

L
Labetalol, 3.36
Lac-operon, 4.45
Lactobacillus, 2.12
Lactose, 4.9
Lactose intolerance, 4.10
Laryngitis, 2.7
Larynx, **5.11**
L-asparaginase, 3.16
Laxatives, **3.56**
LDL, 3.34
LE cell, 1.22
Lead, 1.93, 3.4
Lead poisoning, 4.22

Niemann-Pick disease, 4.20
Nifedipine, 3.24
Nifurtimox, 3.11
Night terrors, 7.6
Nitroglycerin, 3.24
Nitrous oxide, 3.50
Nocardia, 2.19
Non-Hodgkin lymphoma, 1.33, 1.9
Normal flora, **2.3**
NSAIDs, **3.18**
Nucleotides, **4.42**
Null hypothesis, 7.26
Nystagmus, **6.8**
Nystatin, 3.10

O

Observational cohort, **7.27**
Obsessive compulsive, 7.13
Obstructive lung disease, **1.47**
Okazaki fragments, 4.47
Oligoclonal bands, 1.82
Oligodendroblastoma, 1.80
Omeprazole, 3.35
Onchocerca, 2.39
Oncogenes, **1.9**
Oncoviruses, 2.29
Operant conditioning, 7.4
Operator, 4.45
Operon, 4.45
Opiates, 3.4, 7.18, **3.43**
Optic canal, 5.7
Oral contraceptives, 3.41
Orbital fissure, 5.7
Organophosphates, 3.4, 3.37
Orthostasis, 6.28
Osler nodes, 1.44
Osmic acid, 2.2
Osmoregulation, **6.32**
Osmotic diuretics, 3.23
Osteoarthritis, 1.75
Osteoblastoma, 1.78
Osteochondroma, 1.77
Osteogenesis imperfecta, 1.76
Osteoid osteoma, 1.78
Osteoma, 1.78
Osteomalacia, 1.76

Osteomyelitis, 3.6
Osteopetrosis, 1.76
Osteoporosis, 1.76
Osteosarcoma, 1.78
Otitis media, 2.7
Ototoxicity, 3.3
Ovarian tumors, **1.56**
Ovaries, 5.26, **4.34, 4.35**
Ovulation, 6.42
Oxygen binding curve, **6.26**

P

p value, 7.26
p24, 2.30
p53, 1.10
Pacinian corpuscle, 6.6
Paget's disease, 1.59, 1.76
Pain, 1.3
Pancuronium, 3.40
Papilloma, 1.59
Papovavirus, 2.23
Paradoxical cold, 6.6
Paragonimus, 2.37
Parallel play, 7.1
Paraneoplastic syndromes, 1.50
Paranoid personality, 7.12
Parasympathetic ganglia, **5.33**
Parasympathetic nerves, 6.11
Parathyroids, **1.88**
Parietal cells, 6.38
Parkinson's disease, 1.81, **3.51**, 5.34
Parvovirus, 2.23
PAS, 2.2
Passive-aggressive personality, 7.12
Pasteurella, 2.16
Patent ductus arteriosus, 1.39, 1.40
Pedigrees, **1.13**
Pellagra, 4.5
Pelvic fractures, 5.18
Pelvic inflammatory disease, 3.6
Pemphigoid, 1.92
Pemphigus, 1.92
Penicillins, **3.7**
Pentazocine, 3.43
Pentoses, 4.7
Peptic ulcer, **3.35**

Rotor syndrome, 1.69
Roundworms, 2.39
Rubella, 2.25
Rubeola, 2.25

S
Saccharide, **4.9**
Saccharide disorders, **4.10**
Salicylate intoxication, 3.17, 6.24
Salmon patches, 1.92
Salmonella, 2.14
Salt retention, 4.40
Salt wasting, 4.39
Saralasin, 3.21
Scapular winging, 5.12
Scheie syndrome, 4.14
Schilder's disease, 1.82
Schistosoma, 2.37
Schizoid personality, 7.12
Schizophrenia, **7.15**
Schwannoma, 1.80
Scopolamine, 3.39
Scrapie, 2.28
Seborrheic keratosis, 1.91
Secretin, 6.37
Seminoma, 1.55
Senna, 3.55
Sensitivity, **7.21**
Separation anxiety, 7.1
Sepsis, 2.7, 3.6
Sertoli cells, 1.55
Serum sickness, 1.8
Sex hormones, **3.41**
Sexual abuse, 7.19
Sheehan's syndrome, 1.84
Shigella, 2.14
Shingles, 2.24
Shoulder, **5.12**
Sick euthyroid, 1.86
Sickle cell anemia, 1.14, 1.27, 6.25
Side effects, **3.3**
Siderocytes, 1.29
Sigma factor, 4.46
Signal transduction, **6.4**
Sinusitis, 2.7
Sjögren's syndrome, **1.24**

Skeletal muscle, **6.18**
Skin cancer, **1.91**
Skin diseases, **1.92**
Skin infections, 3.10
Skull, **5.7**
SLE, 1.6, 1.20, **1.22**
Sleep apnea, 7.6
Sleep stages, **7.6**
Sleep walking, 7.6
Sleeping sickness, 2.34, 3.11
Slow viral diseases, **2.27**
Smallpox, 2.23, 2.24
Smooth muscle, **6.18**
Somatoform disorders, **7.14**
Somatostatin, 6.37
Somites, 5.1
Specificity, 7.22
Spermatic cord, **5.24**
Spherocytosis, 1.15, 1.27
Sphingolipidoses, 1.14, **4.20**
Sphingolipids, 4.19
Spikes, EEG, 7.17
Spinal shock, 3.38
Spirochetes, **2.20**
Spironolactone, 3.23
Spleen, 1.27
Splitting, 7.5
Spores, 2.4, 2.31
Sporotrichosis, 2.32
Sporozoites, 2.33
Spotted fever, 3.6
Squamous cell carcinoma, 1.91
St. Louis encephalitis, 2.26
Stains, **2.1, 2.2**
Stanford Binet, 7.3
Staphylococci, **2.8**
Staphylococcus aureus, 2.8
Staphylococcus epidermidis, 2.8
Staphylococcus saprophyticus, 2.8
Starch, 4.9
Starry sky pattern, 1.33
Statistics, **7.20**
Status epilepticus, 3.53
Steroids, **4.30**
Stibogluconate, 3.11

Still's disease, 1.75
Stomach, **6.38**
Stool softeners, 3.55
Stranger anxiety, 7.1
Strawberry gallbladder, 1.67
Strawberry hemangiomas, 1.92
Strawberry tongue, 1.60
Strep throat, 2.9
Streptococci, **2.9**
Streptokinase, 3.27
Stretch reflex, 6.16
Striatum, 5.34
Stroke, 5.28
Strongyloides, 2.39
Student's t-test, 7.20
Sturge-Weber, 1.92
Subacromial bursa, 5.12
Subacute sclerosing panencephalitis, 2.27
Succinyl choline, 3.40
Sucralfate, 3.35
Sucrose, 4.9
Sugars, **4.7**
Suicide, **7.7**
Sulfinpyrazone, 3.25
Sulfonylureas, **3.32**
Supination, 5.16
Suramin, 3.11
Sympathetic nerves, 6.11
Syphilis, 1.54, 2.20, 3.6
Syringomyelia, 5.39
Systemic sclerosis, **1.23**

T
Table sugar, 4.9
Taenia solium, 2.38
Takayasu's disease, 1.37
Tapeworms, **2.38**
Tardive dyskinesia, 3.52
Tay-Sachs disease, 4.20
Teichoic acid, 2.4
Tennis elbow, 5.16
Tensilon test, 3.37
Teratoma, 1.54
Terbutaline, 3.30, 3.36
Terfenadine, 3.49
Testes, 5.26

Testes tumors, **1.54**
Testis, **4.32**
Tetanus, 2.13
Tetanus toxin, 2.5
Tetracyclines, 3.13
Thalamus, 5.30, **5.35**
Thalassemias, 1.14, 1.27, 6.25
THC, 3.42
Theca cells, **4.34**
Theophylline, 3.30, 3.46
Thiazides, 3.20, 3.23
Thiopental, 3.48, 3.50
Thromboangiitis obliterans, 1.37
Thromboxane, 3.25
Thrombolytic drugs, **3.27**
Thrush, 1.60
Thyroid, **1.86**
Thyroid tumors, **1.87**
Tibia, fractures, 5.20
Tibial nerve, 5.20
Tinea, 2.32
Tinnitus, 3.17
Tissue plasminogen activator, 3.27
Tolbutamide, 3.32
Tongue, **5.9**
Tonsillitis, 2.7
TORCH, 1.40
Touch receptors, **6.6**
Toxic hepatitis, **1.72**
Toxic shock syndrome toxin, 2.5, 2.8
Toxins, **1.93, 2.5**
Toxoplasma gondii, 2.34, 3.12
Trachoma, 2.21
Traction diverticulum, 1.61
Transcriptase inhibitors, 3.12
Transcription, **4.46**
Transcription factor, 4.45
Transcription, inhibitors of, **3.15**
Transduction, 3.5
Transference, 7.5
Transformation, 3.5
Transient ischemic attacks, **5.29**
Translation, inhibitors of, **3.13**
Transplant rejection, 1.8
Transport, **6.3**

Trazodone, 3.44
Trematodes, **2.37**
Trench fever, 2.22
Treponema pallidum, 1.54, 2.20
Triamterene, 3.23
Triazolam, 3.47
Trichinella, 2.39
Trichomonas, 1.54, **2.36**, 3.6
Tricyclic antidepressants, 3.2, 3.44
Triglycerides, 3.33
Trimeprazine, 3.49
Trimethoprim, 3.14

Trochlear paralysis, 5.8
Tropical sprue, 1.66
Trousseau's sign, 1.35
Trypanosoma, 2.34
Trypsin, 4.3
TTP, 1.26
Tuberculosis, 2.18, 3.6
Tubocurarine, 3.40
Tularemia, 2.16
Tumor markers, **1.11**
Tumor suppressor genes, **1.10**
Turcot's syndrome, 1.64
Type I error, 7.26
Type II error, 7.26
Typhoid fever, 2.14, 3.6
Typhus, 2.22, 3.6
Tyramine, 3.44
Tyrosine kinase, 6.4

U
Ulcerative colitis, 1.20, 1.65
Ulnar nerve, 5.15
Ultimobranchial body, 5.4
Umbilical cord, 5.2
Umbilical ligaments, 5.2
Undoing, 7.5
Undulating fever, 2.16
Upper motor neuron lesions, 1.81
Urachus, 5.2
Ureteric bud, 5.5
Urethritis, 2.7
Urinary tract infection, 3.6
Urogenital development, **5.5**
Urokinase, 3.27

Urolithiasis, **1.53**

V
Valproic acid, 3.53
Variance, 7.20
Vascular tone, 6.13
Vasodilatation, 1.3
Venereal disease, **1.54**
Ventilation, 6.20
Ventricular septal defect, 1.40
Verapamil, 3.24, 3.28
Vertebrobasilar artery, 5.29
Vertigo, 3.54
Viagra, 6.4
Vibrio cholera, 2.15
Vibrio parahaemolyticus, 2.15
Vidarabine, 3.9
Vincristine, 3.16
Vinyl chloride, 1.93
Vioxx, 3.17
Virchow's triad, 1.35
Vitamin K deficiency, 1.26
Vitamins, **4.25**
Vitiligo, 1.92
Volume regulation, **6.32**
Von Gierke's disease, 4.12
Von Recklinghausen's disease, 1.80, 1.92
Von Willebrand disease, 1.15, 1.26
VZV, 2.24

W
Waiter's tip position, 5.14
Waldenström's, 1.34
Wallenberg syndrome, 5.37
Warfarin, 3.26
Warm antibodies, 1.27
Waterhouse-Friderichsen syndrome, 2.10
Weber test, 6.10
WEE, 2.26
Wegener's granulomatosis, 1.6, 1.37, 1.48
Weil-Felix reaction, 2.15
Wernicke, 5.27
Whipple's disease, 1.66, 3.6
Whooping cough, 2.17, 3.6
Wilms' tumor, 3.16
Wilson's disease, 1.73, 5.34

Wiskott-Aldrich syndrome, 1.16, 1.25
Wolff, 5.5
Woolsorter's disease, 2.12
Wrist drop, 5.15
Wuchereria, 2.39

X
Xanthoma, 1.92
X-linked recessive disorders, **1.16**

Y
Yeasts, 2.31
Yellow fever, 2.26
Yersinia pestis, 2.16
Yolk sac, 1.55
Yolk stalk, 5.2

Z
Zenker's diverticulum, 1.61
Ziehl Neelsen stain, 2.2
Zollinger-Ellison syndrome, 1.90, 3.35

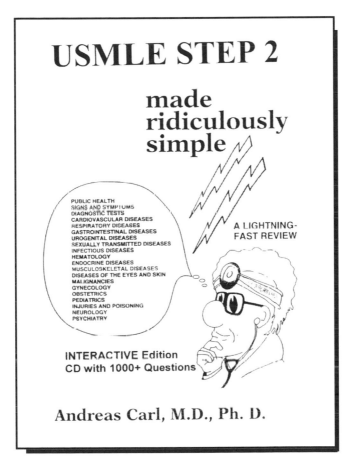

USMLE STEP 2

made ridiculously simple

PUBLIC HEALTH
SIGNS AND SYMPTOMS
DIAGNOSTIC TESTS
CARDIOVASCULAR DISEASES
RESPIRATORY DISEASES
GASTROINTESTINAL DISEASES
UROGENITAL DISEASES
SEXUALLY TRANSMITTED DISEASES
INFECTIOUS DISEASES
HEMATOLOGY
ENDOCRINE DISEASES
MUSCULOSKELETAL DISEASES
DISEASES OF THE EYES AND SKIN
MALIGNANCIES
GYNECOLOGY
OBSTETRICS
PEDIATRICS
INJURIES AND POISONING
NEUROLOGY
PSYCHIATRY

A LIGHTNING-FAST REVIEW

INTERACTIVE Edition
CD with 1000+ Questions

Andreas Carl, M.D., Ph. D.

384 pages - 275 charts

♦ Systematic Review of Diseases and Organ Systems in Chart Format

♦ Patient Management and Therapy

♦ Easy to Memorize !!!

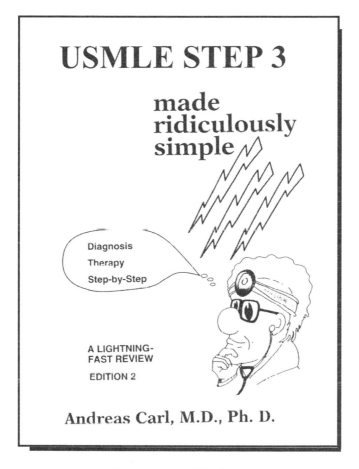

USMLE STEP 3

made ridiculously simple

Diagnosis
Therapy
Step-by-Step

A LIGHTNING-
FAST REVIEW

EDITION 2

Andreas Carl, M.D., Ph. D.

312 pages   -   395 charts

♦ Step-by-Step Approach (*"What do you do next?"*)

♦ Ideal Preparation for Computer Case Simulations

♦ Easy to Memorize !!!